COVID-19, INEQUALITY AND OLDER PEOPLE

Everyday Life during the Pandemic

Camilla Lewis, Chris Phillipson, Sophie Yarker
and Luciana Lang

With a foreword by
Andy Burnham

P

First published in Great Britain in 2023 by

Policy Press, an imprint of
Bristol University Press
University of Bristol
1–9 Old Park Hill
Bristol
BS2 8BB
UK
t: +44 (0)117 374 6645
e: bup-info@bristol.ac.uk

Details of international sales and distribution partners are available at
policy.bristoluniversitypress.co.uk

British Library Cataloguing in Publication Data
A catalogue record for this book is available from the British Library

ISBN 978-1-4473-6744-4 paperback
ISBN 978-1-4473-6745-1 ePub
ISBN 978-1-4473-6746-8 OA Pdf

Cover design: Nicky Borowiec
Front cover image: Adobe Stock/John

Contents

List of figures and tables

Figures

Tables

About the authors

Camilla Lewis is Lecturer in Architectural Studies at the University of Manchester. Her research centres on the themes of urban change, inequalities, housing, ageing, belonging and community. Her work has a strong methodological focus, spanning a variety of ethnographic, sensory as well as longitudinal approaches. Her publications provide theoretical analyses on the everyday experiences of inequalities in urban environments and also practical suggestions for how to tackle marginalisation in socially excluded groups.

Chris Phillipson is Professor of Sociology and Social Gerontology at the University of Manchester. He has published widely on issues relating to critical gerontology, social exclusion in later life, and the development of age-friendly cities and communities.

Sophie Yarker is Research Fellow in Sociology at the University of Manchester. She has a background in both sociology and human geography and research interests in urban neighbourhoods, social infrastructure, ageing in place and local belonging and identities. Her current research explores age-friendly policy and experiences of ageing in place in cities.

Luciana Lang is Research Associate at the University of Manchester. She works in socio-ecological anthropology in urban contexts. She is interested in community use of the commons, from mangroves to pocket parks. Her research on the impact of COVID-19 on older people has revealed the crucial role of green spaces and social infrastructure in later life and across different ethnic and identity groups.

Acknowledgements

The authors are extremely grateful to the large number of people and organisations who provided support and advice through the various phases of the study. The research is built around the experiences of 21 organisations across Greater Manchester, together with interviews with 102 people aged 50 and over living in various neighbourhoods across the region. The research team is hugely grateful for their willingness to talk about the impact of COVID-19.

The study would not have been possible without the support of Christine Oliver, Senior Evidence Manager, Centre for Ageing Better (CfAB), Nicola Waterworth, Greater Manchester Partnership Manager (CfAB), and Dave Thorley, Programme Lead, Age-Friendly Manchester, at Manchester City Council, all of whom responded with speed and enthusiasm to requests for funding at different phases of the project. We are also grateful to the following: John Hannen, Programme Manager, Ambition for Ageing, for his consistent support and for securing a grant through the National Lottery Community Fund's Ageing Better Programme; Atiha Chaudry, Chair of Manchester BME Network, for co-ordinating the involvement of community-based organisations which allowed the research to engage with sections of the South Asian community in Greater Manchester; Charles Kwaku-Odio of the Caribbean and African Health Network who also provided important contacts with the African Caribbean community in Greater Manchester; and Marie Greenhalgh, Founder Director of Wythenshawe Good Neighbours, for her valuable advice at different stages of the work. The project also received excellent advice and support from Paul McGarry, Assistant Director, Public Service Reform Directorate, Greater Manchester Combined Authority.

We would like to thank members of the Manchester Urban Ageing Research Group, in particular, Tine Buffel, Patty Doran and Mhorag Goff, for carrying out interviews and being involved in the wider project exploring the impact of COVID-19 on older people living in Greater Manchester. We are also very appreciative of the fine work of Katayha Gould in producing illustrations for the book. Lastly, we would like to thank the Centre for Ageing Better, and the University of the Manchester, Faculty of Humanities Social Responsibility fund, for financial support for Open Access.

Foreword

Andy Burnham
Mayor of Greater Manchester

The onset of the COVID-19 pandemic in March 2020 will have amplified alarm bells already sounding in some communities across Greater Manchester. COVID-19 exposed, and in many cases widened, the already deep divisions that existed in society. Places and communities already experiencing inequalities in health and finances – so often in the North – were hit harder than others, and the uncertainty and insecurity affecting many people's livelihoods and well-being was laid bare.

In Greater Manchester, rates of mortality from COVID-19 were 25 per cent higher than in England as a whole. More than a quarter of deaths, in the first wave of the pandemic, were among people living in the most deprived communities of the region. The higher COVID-19 infection and death rates experienced by people in our Bangladeshi, Pakistani and Black communities can in large part be explained by the various inequalities experienced by these groups. In the summer of 2020, we all shared in the anguish and frustration about the racism and discrimination that blights the lives of too many of our residents.

The period since the onset of the pandemic has proved immensely difficult for many, and particularly for those suffering from low-waged, precarious employment, and a decline in the value of benefits. But neighbourhoods and individuals – as this book shows – demonstrated remarkable resilience throughout the COVID-19 crisis. We must adopt the same determination when it comes forging a recovery that puts us in a stronger, fairer and more resilient position. This can be a moment of real change, and now is the time to seize it. As a Greater Manchester family, we must put tackling inequality – exposed like never before by COVID-19 – at the heart of our response to the challenges we now face.

This book provides a powerful account of how the daily lives of older people were affected by COVID-19. It highlights the variety of responses from groups and neighbourhoods across the city-region. It documents, as well, the important work of voluntary and community organisations and the crucial role which they played in providing support to vulnerable groups. The book also makes a compelling case for working directly with communities, both in preventing another pandemic and addressing the injustices exposed by COVID-19.

In some ways, the ruptures of the pandemic presented us with a chance to speed up the delivery of our ambitions for Greater Manchester. In undertaking this task, the book offers a timely reminder of the importance of community-based work. True 'levelling up' cannot just be about promises of infrastructure in the distant future. It must be about the issues currently affecting people's lives, their homes and their neighbourhoods – securing real improvement in the areas which have a direct impact on the quality of daily life.

We are proud that Greater Manchester is the UK's first Age-Friendly City-Region as recognised by the World Health Organization. This is a fantastic achievement and a testament to the hard work of so many people. But we need to keep taking practical steps to make changes for all groups of older people, and to make sure that we are living not just extended years but happier and healthier lives.

We want to help bring about a city-region that works for everyone, where the economy serves the people, and where everyone has a voice. As this book makes clear, this includes supporting older people in their neighbourhoods, listening to what they have to say about the issues affecting them, and involving people directly in planning for the future.

We have always been clear that the diversity and the vibrancy of our city-region is our greatest strength. All our communities have something to give and something to gain from working together. We want to improve the lives of older people in Greater Manchester, so that residents are able to contribute to – and benefit from – sustained prosperity, and enjoy a good quality of life. This book highlights some of the challenges that we will have to overcome, but charts a path that will help us to get there together.

1

Introduction

In the period since early 2020, SARS-CoV-2 (COVID-19) developed into one of the deadliest infectious diseases of the last one hundred years. The arrival of the virus presented an international crisis, the universality of which has rarely been seen within recent history (Whitehead and Torossian, 2021). As the pandemic evolved, it came to represent far more than just a global health problem, but one which affected a broad range of social, cultural and economic institutions. Few areas of everyday life were left 'unchanged in the wake of the emergence of this new infectious disease' (Lupton and Willis, 2021: 4). To avoid infection, or infecting others, people were required to learn new social behaviours, such as wearing face masks, washing their hands more frequently, maintaining physical distance from others outside their households, staying at home as much as possible, and avoiding gathering in groups. For an extended period, daily life was disrupted in many significant ways, its varied impacts continuing to affect groups and societies across the Global North and South (Horton, 2021).

COVID-19 created new pressures for people of all ages throughout the world but raised particular concern for *older age groups*. This was especially the case for those living alone, those from marginalised backgrounds, people with long-standing illnesses, and individuals living in communities affected by high levels of deprivation. As Sugrue has argued:

> Just as COVID-19 is particularly dangerous to populations with pre-existing conditions, the virus ferociously swept across the world because of pre-existing social conditions: the precarity of work; the unaffordability of housing; the depth of racial, ethnic and class divides; a profoundly unequal global economy; and the failure of many governments worldwide to rise to the challenges. (Sugrue, 2022: 1)

Strategies to control COVID-19 led to various forms of exclusion affecting all age groups, but raised particular issues for older people, for example, around the effects of social distancing, digital exclusion, loss of access to community support and social isolation (Walsh et al, 2021).

Despite the burgeoning literature on the pandemic, there remain few detailed accounts of *everyday life* under COVID-19 (though see Garthwaite and Patrick, 2022, for an important collection on children and families) and the enduring pressures facing particular groups within the older population.

As yet, little is known about the extent to which social distancing measures disrupted older adults' social connections during the pandemic, and the resulting consequences for everyday life (Fuller and Huseth-Zosel, 2022; Vlachantoni et al, 2022). The *social dimensions* of the pandemic were often marginalised in research and debate, for reasons identified in Chapter 2. However, such dimensions are crucial to consider, as social variables will be highly influential in shaping both the medium- and long-term outcomes of the pandemic. In this context, Christakis makes the point that '[f]or the elderly, the chronically ill, the poor, the imprisoned, and the socially marginalized, the SARS-2 pandemic might continue to be a biological threat long after the majority of the population has moved on psychologically and practically and long after overall levels of the virus are low' (2020: 318).

The aim of this book is to provide a contribution to understanding the social dimensions of the COVID-19 crisis. It draws upon novel *qualitative longitudinal research* which recorded the experiences of a diverse group of people aged 50 and over, in a variety of situations and locations across Greater Manchester (GM), England. The women and men were interviewed over three 'lockdowns', covering a 12-month period of the pandemic. The analysis explores the strategies they adopted to minimise the effect of COVID-19 on their lives, and the extent to which social distancing created new vulnerabilities for some of those interviewed. In doing this, an important aim of the book is to *advance sociological understanding* about the effect of COVID-19, both on older people as well as the social networks of which they are a part.

The interviews reveal how daily life changed under the various lockdowns over the course of 2020 and early 2021, and how older people made sense of the changes affecting their lives and relationships. The analysis explores the variations in these responses, focusing in particular on ethnic minority people, those living in lower-income neighbourhoods, and those from the lesbian, gay, bisexual, transgender, queer and other (LGBTQ+) community. Our findings indicate that while many older people experienced a decline in social contact during the pandemic, others responded by developing new relationships, as well as drawing on existing social networks. The book argues that the pandemic is likely to have a long-term impact on the way certain people think about their health and well-being, their use of shared spaces, and their social relationships more generally.

The impact of the pandemic on older people

Older people were disproportionately affected by the emergence and spread of COVID-19, whether in hospital, the community or in care homes (Sachs et al, 2022). The United Nations Economic Commission for Europe

(UNECE) described how the pandemic had 'particularly grave implications' for older people across all countries of the Global North and South (2022: 6). In the case of England and Wales, in 2020 the mortality rate from COVID-19 at age 80–84 was 6.5 times higher than at ages 65–69 and 57 times higher than at ages under 65 (Raleigh, 2022). Raleigh comments that:

> Covid-19 changed the health profile of England's population radically by becoming the leading cause of death in 2020 and 2021. The number of people dying from Covid-19 exceeded the number of people dying from the most common killers in preceding years (eg, dementia and Alzheimer's disease, heart disease, stroke and lung cancer). (Raleigh, 2022)

Estimates from the World Health Organization (2022) of the full death toll associated directly or indirectly with the COVID-19 pandemic (described as 'excess mortality') for the period 1 January 2020 to 31 December 2021 suggest 14.9 million deaths, with the majority of these clustered in the older age groups. The scale of the disaster affecting older people is illustrated by figures from the United States. Over the period January 2020 to September, 2022, 1,004,760 deaths were recorded from COVID-19, of which 973,896 (that is, over 90 per cent) were among people aged 50 and over, with 542,795 deaths among those aged 75 and over (Statista, 2022).

Rules based around age-based restrictions were introduced in numerous countries, instructing older people to quarantine for prolonged periods and avoid contact with others (Corley et al, 2021). Such rules represented 'state intervention of extraordinary severity, within a broader context of cataclysmic global events' (Fletcher, 2021: 480). In the United Kingdom, in March 2020, the government advised all people aged 70 and above to self-isolate for a minimum of 12 weeks. Guidelines were based on evidence that COVID-19 severity was strongly age-associated, with older people being at greater risk, compared with other groups, of hospitalisation and death.

A number of studies have highlighted a range of negative outcomes of the pandemic and social distancing rules on older people, including mental health problems (Settersten et al, 2020), loss of connections with friends and family (Portacolone et al, 2021), and a rise in ageism and intergenerational tensions (Ayalon et al, 2021; see Chapter 2, this volume). The pandemic has had in fact numerous and serious consequences for a range of social groups, for example, women, young adults, those living alone, people of lower educational attainment, and people with learning disabilities (Courtney and Cooper, 2021; Fancourt et al, 2022). Such findings illustrate that the implications of COVID-19 are 'myriad, far-reaching, and unanticipated, making it critical to examine what effects stay-at-home orders, mandated social distancing, and a possible loss of social connections may have on the health and well-being of already vulnerable, socially isolated individuals' (Bundy et al, 2021: 874).

An important debate within the research literature concerns the extent to which events such as COVID-19 may exacerbate feelings of loneliness and social isolation among groups such as older adults (Bundy et al, 2021; Kim and Jung, 2021; Macdonald and Hülür, 2021). While definitions vary, loneliness is generally perceived as a subjective and unpleasant emotional state, whereas social isolation is defined as an objective or factual state that infers absence of contact with other people (Willis et al, 2022). This book pays particular attention to the way in which social contacts changed over the period of study, and the extent to which this affected social relationships among our participants.

The research provides one of the few detailed accounts of how older people's everyday lives changed over the course of three successive lockdowns, which were designed to manage the spread of the virus. The following questions are addressed: *How did older people's everyday lives change over this period? What kinds of support did older people draw upon? How did social distancing affect relationships and contacts within neighbourhoods?*

Background to the study

As concerns about COVID-19 increased in the early spring of 2020, the project team worked with their existing networks across GM to plan a programme of community-based research to assess possible social consequences arising from the pandemic (Phillipson et al, 2021). The research team are all members of the Manchester Urban Ageing Research Group (MUARG), which brings together scholars from different disciplines to identify new ways of responding to the challenges associated with population ageing in urban environments. The aim of the group's research is to understand the relationship between population ageing and urban change, a theme which has become a major issue for public policy and an increasingly important area for interdisciplinary research. By 2030, two-thirds of the world's populations will be living in cities, with major urban areas in the developed world likely to have 25 per cent or more of their population aged 60 and over (Buffel et al, 2018). This study takes the example of GM, a major urban region in the UK, and explores the impact of COVID-19 on its socially diverse neighbourhoods.

MUARG members have been involved in a range of projects over the past two decades, developing innovative research on the lives of older people living in areas of multiple deprivation (see Yarker, 2022b). Much of this research has been conducted in partnership with older people living in low-income neighbourhoods across GM (and other regions in Europe), and with local authorities, voluntary organisations and community groups.

Building on their existing networks, the project team worked closely with community organisations involved in supporting older people during the pandemic. As the book highlights, COVID-19 exposed areas of strength, creativity and innovation among various community and mutual aid groups (see also British Academy, 2021). For older people themselves, there were a variety of reactions to the pandemic. Few of those interviewed were left untouched by its profound effects on the routines and relationships which comprise daily life. The aim of the book is to convey the challenges and responses across the different organisations and groups of older people interviewed, examining both the impact of social distancing and the various responses which emerged.

Working across the city-region, the project team formed a network of community organisations to assist with the study. A *Research Advisory Board* was established, consisting of stakeholders who worked with older people from a range of neighbourhoods and backgrounds (see Chapter 3). The board provided guidance on each part of the research process, including the recruitment of participants, the format for the interviews and the dissemination of findings. The research team is indebted to all those who gave their time to talk about their experiences. We hope that this book will prove valuable in developing policies to support communities and organisations in the varied tasks to aid the recovery from the pandemic.

Interdisciplinary approach and aims

The book takes a novel approach, exploring detailed narratives of older people's experiences of the pandemic, using what is known as a *longitudinal perspective*, which included interviewing the same individual(s) at different points in time. This method enabled the project team to explore the everyday lives of older people from a multidimensional perspective, ranging from studying the influence of experiences over the life-course, to the role of the individual's social network in providing help and support. The research also emphasised the importance of viewing the study of everyday life as an 'interdisciplinary endeavour' (Hall, 2019). In this study, drawing on the anthropological, geographical and sociological backgrounds of the research team.

Based upon an initial literature review, and on prior experiences of working with older age groups in GM, a number of research questions were identified as central for developing an understanding of the impact of the pandemic. These were:

- How do older people at risk of social exclusion experience 'social distancing'?
- How has social distancing affected everyday life and support networks?
- What capacities and resources (individual or community level) do older people draw on when negotiating the experience of social distancing?

- What has been the impact of social distancing over time?
- What types of support services exist or could be developed to alleviate the impact of social distancing on older people experiencing exclusion and isolation?

The book develops an *interdisciplinary approach* to understanding the unequal impact of COVID-19 across the older population. The analysis brings together theoretical approaches to the life-course, everyday life, home-making and relationships (from sociology and anthropology), with analytical tools for understanding ageing and caring responsibilities (from gerontology and geography). Theoretical tools from geography and urban studies were also used to explore the interrelationship between spatial and social inequalities. Bringing together these different approaches enables a better understanding of the impact of the pandemic on older people, the organisations working on their behalf and the communities in which they live.

Outline of the chapters

The chapters are structured as follows: Chapter 2 provides a sociological analysis of the COVID-19 pandemic, with reference to the *social context* affecting ageing populations, together with the impact of the pandemic on different groups of older people. Although the effect of COVID-19 has been examined in various ways, its broad social and cultural determinants have been given much less consideration in research. The chapter outlines a theoretical framework for understanding the pressures facing older people in the context of the emergence of what is viewed as a more 'precarious' society.

Following on from this discussion, Chapter 3 outlines the *methodology* used in the study, explaining how a qualitative longitudinal approach was used in order to capture the experiences of older people over a 12-month period of the pandemic. Details about the sample, recruitment and data analysis are presented, as well as reflections about the opportunities and limitations of working during the pandemic. The chapter also provides information about the GM region, which provided the location for interviews with older people and community organisations.

The following four chapters report on the *research findings*. Chapter 4 examines the *everyday lives of older people during the pandemic*, discussing changes affecting people's lives over the period of data collection. Drawing upon the views and experiences reported by our participants, the following themes are discussed: the impact of shielding; social distancing and social isolation; growing old under lockdown; and reflections on the impact of COVID-19.

Focusing on *four case studies*, Chapter 5 explores how experiences of the pandemic differed greatly between individuals, depending on their biographies and daily lives prior to the pandemic. The findings reveal how biographical *turning points* affected responses and experiences to the pandemic.

Building on these findings, Chapter 6 explores how *social and caring relationships* were reorientated during lockdown, what impact this had on older people, and what factors were behind the various changes. The analysis is organised around five themes: *increased social isolation*; *pressures at home*; *changes in contact with neighbours and in the neighbourhood*; *the role of outdoor spaces*; and *the role of technology*. To analyse experiences of contracting and expanding social worlds, a theoretical framework known as *landscapes of care* is used. This considers the different spaces through which caring relationships were experienced, as well as the different spatial patterns that emerged due to social distancing.

The focus of Chapter 7 is on the interviews carried out with 21 *community-based organisations* (including mutual-aid groups, voluntary bodies, neighbourhood groups, faith-based groups) in GM during the pandemic. The discussion examines the role these organisations played in responding to the pandemic and how their responses changed over the 12-month period. The analysis considers the critical role of social infrastructure (libraries, community centres) in providing support to older people, and the consequences arising from cuts to facilities over the period since 2010. The findings are analysed in relation to broader discussion about the precarity faced by both older people and the organisations providing support within the community.

Drawing together the themes outlined in the preceding four chapters, Chapter 8 presents a *discussion* of some of the cross–cutting issues which arose across the empirical chapters. It focuses on two main elements of our findings: *general experiences of daily life under the pandemic* and *issues and concerns relevant to the future care and support of older people*.

Considering these findings further, Chapter 9 makes recommendations for policy with links to the World Health Organization's 'Age–Friendly Cities' initiative, which has been influential in raising awareness about the need to adapt urban environments to the demands of ageing populations. A combination of widening inequalities within and between urban environments, and the impact of austerity on local government and city budgets, has raised questions about future progress in developing age-friendly programmes and related activities (Buffel et al, 2018). These pressures have been compounded by the impact of COVID-19. Considering this context, the discussion outlines a number of recommendations in relation to developing a '*community-centred approach*' in responding to future variants of COVID-19, as well as making suggestions for how to create a post-pandemic urban environment.

The Conclusion draws together the main themes of the book, highlighting the challenges older people faced when forced to 'stay apart' from family and friends, and identifies changes affecting people over time through three successive lockdowns. The authors call for greater attention to the impact of the pandemic on older people, to counter negative social attitudes towards ageing where the older population are increasingly presented as a burden on communities. The discussion also suggests that the policy concepts of 'age-friendly' and 'ageing in place' must be updated with a deeper understanding of the changing conditions of daily life for older people brought about by COVID-19.

Overall, this book offers a novel analysis of the ways in which COVID-19 has exposed and exacerbated inequalities in ageing (see also Buffel et al, 2021). Our analysis supports Portacolone et al's (2021) argument that COVID-19 *amplified* existing insecurities, as people struggled to cope with long-term illnesses in the context of pressures from reduced health and social care support. Extending this argument further, our findings also suggest that the pandemic has *introduced new vulnerabilities*, exacerbating further the precarious lives of some groups of older people.

The book includes illustrations by Katayha Gould, based on extracts from the interviews, to represent key points. Illustrations have been used in other social science research studies, as a way of depicting key findings (Heath et al, 2018). Drawings or images offer a helpful way of conveying emotion, providing a description and capturing a scene or situation (Hammond and Wellington, 2021). The aim of including illustrations is to enliven the research data, making the lived experiences of the participants compelling and accessible. The research team worked closely with Katayha to devise illustrations which depict particular moments described by the participants in the interviews. These images are, of course, interpretations based on the project team's analysis of the findings and Katayha's artistic interpretation of these events.

2

A sociological analysis of the impact of COVID-19 on older people

Introduction

This chapter provides a sociological analysis of the COVID-19 pandemic, with reference to the demographic and social contexts influencing ageing populations, and the impact of the pandemic on different groups of older people. Although the effects of COVID-19 have been examined in various ways, its broad social and cultural determinants have been given much less consideration in research. Indeed, as will be argued further, one result of the pandemic has been to greatly strengthen approaches which view ageing from a biomedical perspective, marginalising the broader cultural, economic and social forces which influence later life.

Grenier and Phillipson (2023) argue that the emergency conditions of the pandemic have increased the power of biomedicine and its influence over the lives of older people. Prior to COVID-19, the experiences of older people requiring access to health and care were already heavily medicalised through assessments of function and/or cognition (Grenier et al, 2020). It is thus not surprising that a group already subjected to disease-based models and health practices found these reinforced in a variety of ways as a result of the conditions imposed by COVID-19. In contrast, the aim of this book, as outlined in Chapter 1, is to explore the social construction and social consequences of the pandemic associated with COVID-19. Following Bonilla, the pandemic should be seen as 'a socially produced event, driven not by biological forces or natural hazards, but by the deeply rooted social inequalities that shape our experiences of those hazards to begin with' (2022: 420). Bonilla further argues that: 'The truth is that the pandemic is a disaster in the sociological sense: a sudden catastrophic event but also a revelation of failures, an episode that exacerbates already existing inequalities, and a moment of reckoning' (2022: 424).

Similarly, Horton makes the point that:

> The coronavirus has hit societies weakened by political and economic forces that have been at work for generations. The inequalities that have deepened in recent years have worsened the risks of COVID-19. Unless governments devise policies and programmes that reverse these

profound disparities, our societies will never be COVID-19 secure. (Horton, 2021: 20–21)

Such inequalities, interacting with COVID-19 and equivalent disasters, have and will continue to have a dramatic effect on the lives of older people. The devastating toll of lives lost – 'premature mortality' in more neutral scientific language – has still to be accounted for, especially with regards to its impact on family and community networks (see Chapter 4). The lengthy absence of access to the normal rituals associated with mourning (or contact with those dying) has been one important concern. Harrop et al (2020) found that over the period from spring to autumn 2020, 85 per cent of people experiencing a bereavement were unable to say goodbye to their loved one in a way in which they would have chosen. But in a more general way, the dominance of the biomedical over the social has limited our understanding of the way life changed during the pandemic. Lives certainly became more vulnerable or 'precarious' but what did this mean for how people managed everyday life, especially those experiencing insecurity even before the pandemic took hold?

This chapter puts forward a sociological framework for understanding the implications of the pandemic on older people. The first part outlines the background to the dominance of biomedical interpretations of COVID-19, and the implications for understanding the lives of older people. Second, the chapter examines in more detail the uneven effects of the pandemic, with a particular focus on ethnic minority groups, and those living in lower-income neighbourhoods. Finally, the chapter draws the arguments together by putting forward a theoretical framework for understanding the pressures facing older people in the context of a more 'precarious' society (Grenier et al, 2020).

Biomedical constructions of ageing

In their classic essay analysing the 'dangers and dilemmas' associated with what they term the 'biomedicalization of aging', Estes and Binney identify two related features of this phenomena: '(1) the social construction of aging in terms of a medical problem (thinking of aging as a medical problem) and (2) the praxis (or practice) of aging as a medical problem (behaviours and policies growing out of thinking about aging as a medical problem)' (1989: 587). A key feature for Estes and Binney was the way in which the dominance of the medical model in approaches to ageing 'took precedence over, and in many cases defines, the basic biological, social and behavioural processes and problems of aging' (1989: 589).

The argument developed in this chapter is that 'thinking of ageing' as a medical problem was strengthened considerably as the COVID-19 pandemic unfolded. As a form of practice, it became the dominant approach in framing our understanding of how to respond generally to COVID-19, and to older people in particular. Again, to quote Estes and Binney: 'The biomedical has become the "institutionalized thought structure" of the field, despite increasing evidence of the importance of social and behavioural factors in explaining health and aging' (1989: 589).

But why, it might be argued, is this a problem? Surely, in a pandemic (and especially in a crisis of the kind experienced with COVID-19) we need precisely the insights and expertise associated with the disciplines linked with biomedicine. Indeed, it is important to emphasise the significant gains made through innovations associated with the development of vaccines which had such a dramatic effect in controlling and reducing the effect of various waves of the pandemic (Farrar, 2021; Gilbert and Green, 2021; Sridhar, 2022). Yet the dominance of biomedicine in the context of COVID-19 has led to a number of problems in respect of the treatment of older people. These are reflected in, first, the lack of awareness or refusal to confront the implications of the huge toll of deaths skewed towards the older age groups; second, the presentation of older people as a homogeneous and vulnerable group; third, and linked with both, the consolidation of ageist attitudes towards older people during the pandemic.

The first of these is perhaps the most surprising – and in some respects most worrying. Statistics about deaths from COVID-19 are indeed difficult to grasp in their enormity – 14.9 million excess deaths according to the World Health Organization, as noted in Chapter 1, for the period up to December 2021 (other studies cite an even higher figure for the same time period, see Wang et al, 2022). At any age, a death is important – a grievous loss to a family and community somewhere in the world. But do we make sufficient notice of the fact that the majority of these were indeed older people – some in their 50s and 60s but most in their 70s and beyond? Is the word 'excess deaths' itself a problem when applied to an event such as COVID-19? These are deaths over and above what would have been expected in the absence of a pandemic. However, in the rush to feel a sense of triumph over the achievement of controlling the pandemic (at least in the Global North), the fact that we have lost a substantial group who may have lived for five, ten or even 20 or more years within their communities has been glossed over. Does the absence of a discussion about this indicate that death on a mass scale is difficult for societies to talk about or make sense of? Or is it the fact that it is indeed mainly older people and hence their deaths were in some sense 'understandable' or 'might have happened anyway'?

The avoidance of discussing the scale of death and long-term illness among older people as a result of COVID-19 has been facilitated by two other factors linked to the influence of biomedicine. First, the pandemic reinforced a narrative of older people as predominantly frail and vulnerable, one which 'conflated chronological age with impairment, incompetence, but also helplessness' (Swift and Chasteen, 2021: 249). The vulnerability narrative is problematic because it emphasises the similarities rather than the differences between older adults, as well as ignoring the significant positions they occupy within communities. Contrary to the stereotype of vulnerability, evidence suggests that older adults made vital contributions in alleviating problems during the pandemic, as caregivers, volunteers operating helplines, assisting children with their homework remotely, or by returning to work in the case of retired health-care workers (World Health Organization, 2021). Gullette (1997) refers to the tendency to depict experiences of ageing according to impairment and loss as part of a 'decline narrative', a characteristic which was substantially reinforced as the pandemic unfolded over the course of 2020.

The emphasis on vulnerability was itself part of a wider problem which emerged early in the pandemic, namely, the reinforcement of ageism and age discrimination, illustrated in important areas of health and public policy affecting older people. Kendall-Taylor et al (2020) describe how the pandemic pushed cultural bias against older people to new heights in the United States, framing older people as a monolithic group, failing to acknowledge their demographic, health and functional diversity. Ayalon and colleagues outline the issues in the following terms:

> [W]ith the pandemic there has been a parallel outbreak of ageism. What we are seeing in public discourse is an increasing portrayal of those over the age of 70 as being all alike with regard to being helpless, frail, and unable to contribute to society. These views are being spread by the social media, the press, and public announcements by government officials throughout the world. (Ayalon et al, 2021: e49)

Ageism was evident even at the start of the pandemic, as illustrated by the crisis which unfolded in residential and nursing home care across Europe and North America. Care settings took a disproportionate toll of deaths in the various waves of the virus – around 40 per cent in the first wave for the UK, with a similar figure for the United States (Gullette, 2022); and around 25 per cent for the second and third waves in the UK (Curry, 2021). Taking a measure of excess deaths (that is, deaths above the expected number for any given period) raises the figure even higher: in the case of the UK, from 19,286 deaths between mid-March and mid-June 2020 in residential care homes where the virus was mentioned on the death certificate, to 35,067 excess deaths registered in the same period (Curry, 2021). Williams et al (2022) calculate a 79 per cent increase in deaths in care homes in England and Wales in the first two months of the pandemic in 2020. This was a period when care homes were largely 'abandoned' in the first wave of COVID-19 with the transferring of untested older people from hospitals into care homes, the withdrawal of inspections by the Care Quality Commission, and restrictions on access to hospitals for residents in care settings (Health Foundation, cited in Calvert and Arbuthnot, 2021). Moreover, 'pre-existing conditions' affecting care homes increased the likelihood of deaths at the level experienced, with homes (in England) going into the crisis with 40 per cent annual staff turnover, 122,000 staff vacancies and 25 per cent of workers on zero-hour contracts.

Gullette describes a similar crisis pre-COVID-19 in the US context:

> Pre-coronavirus, Medicaid [a programme designed to assist low-income households with health care expenses] rates dropped too low to cover costs, and facilities kept wages too low and aides' hours too short for them to provide adequate sufficient care. Many facilities failed state tests for adequate infection programmes – failures ignored by the agencies responsible for monitoring them. In 2017, the Trump administration reduced the fines against nursing homes for harming patients, even when this harm resulted in a resident's death. (Gullette, 2022: 239)

Ageism was also a factor in determining whether older people with COVID-19 got access to hospital care and the type of treatment they received. This was illustrated in a study by Calvert and Arbuthnot (2021) of Britain's response to the pandemic crisis. During the first wave of the pandemic, 47,000 people died of COVID-19, but only around 5,000 received the top level of critical care. At the peak of the first wave, just 2.5 per cent of patients in intensive care were over the age of 80. The authors conclude that many hospitals used some form of triage to restrict intensive care for those 60 and over. From examination of data (for England and Wales) of people admitted to intensive care units, Calvert and Arbuthnot found that:

> The majority of those who died without the highest level of life-saving care were the oldest patients. More than half of those who died of the virus in hospital during the first wave were aged over 80 and yet only 2.5 percent of patients in that age group were admitted to critical care. If they had been given intensive care, they might have survived. In the few cases where patients over 80 were given intensive care to treat the virus, 38 percent were discharged alive during the first wave of the outbreak. (Calvert and Arbuthnot, 2021: 251)

It is difficult to avoid the conclusion that 'thinking of older people as medical problems' became a significant obstacle to providing equitable treatment in care settings such as hospitals and nursing homes. And it is difficult as well not to conclude that:

> [M]illions of deaths among [older people] could have been prevented if societies valued care work. Instead in those countries which warehouse the elderly and infirm in nursing and retirement homes, care workers

are chronically underpaid and overworked and often uninsured, susceptible to infection but unable to miss work even when they fall ill. (Sugrue, 2022: 5)

But it is also the case that many died because of the way in which the COVID-19 crisis interacted with a National Health Service (NHS) which was itself weakened through a decade of austerity, with reductions in staffing levels, low pay, and increased waiting lists for appointments and operations. Davis concludes that:

> The Government's deficit reduction policies ... resulted in a slowing down, and in some cases, a reversal of social progress made in the previous decade. As a result, health gains slowed, stopped or even reversed and this affected lower income groups in particular. The increase in health inequalities meant that when the pandemic struck, the vulnerable in society suffered to a disproportionate degree. (Davis, 2022: 47)

Indeed, what has been highlighted by the pandemic is precisely the dangers associated with an 'institutionalised thought structure' which neglects the importance of social and behavioural factors in the determination of ill-health. What this meant in practical terms was the lack of preparation for precisely the uneven distribution of the impact of COVID-19, with ethnic minority and low-income communities among the worst to suffer from the effects of the pandemic.

COVID-19 and social inequality

This section examines the uneven distribution of the COVID-19 pandemic, with particular emphasis on ethnic minority communities and areas characterised by multiple deprivation. Between 8 December 2020 (the start of the vaccination programme) and 12 June 2021 (the approximate end of the second wave of the pandemic), people from all ethnic minority groups (except the Chinese group and women in the White other ethnic group) experienced higher rates of death involving COVID-19 compared with the White British population (ONS, 2022a). During this period, the rate of death involving COVID-19 was highest for the Bangladeshi ethnic group (five times greater than the White British group for males, and 4.5 times greater for females), followed by the Pakistani (3.1 for males, 2.6 for females) and Black African (2.4 for males, 1.7 for females) ethnic groups (ONS, 2022a). Men and women from Black Caribbean and Black African backgrounds continued to be at elevated risk in the third wave after adjusting for location, measures of disadvantage, occupation, living arrangements, pre-existing health conditions, and after vaccination status is taken into account (ONS, 2022a).

Nazroo and Bécares (2021) argue that inequalities in relation to COVID-19 and ethnic minority people are the result of pre-existing social and economic inequalities manifesting in the form of particular chronic illnesses. The authors conclude that: 'The inequalities that are faced by ethnic minority people are driven by entrenched structural and institutional racism and racial discrimination … leading to their disproportionate representation in insecure and low-paid employment, overcrowded housing, and deprived neighbourhoods' (Nazroo and Bécares, 2021: 2).

People from Pakistani and Bangladeshi communities are more likely to be involved in work that carries risk of exposure to the virus (such as retail, hospitality, taxi driving) and to live in households which amplify disadvantage, due to higher numbers of multigenerational family members with chronic, disabling illnesses (ONS, 2022b). Pakistani and Bangladeshi groups are also more likely to be living with two or more health conditions which interact to produce a greater risk of death from COVID-19 (ONS, 2022b). Compared with their White British counterparts, estimates of disability-free life expectancy are approximately ten years lower for Bangladeshi men and 12 years lower for Pakistani women (Watkinson et al, 2021).

Compared to people from other backgrounds, these groups are also more likely to reside in deprived areas (Nafiliyn et al, 2021). Drawing on data from the UK Biobank, Razieh et al (2021) examined the extent to which the excess risk of testing positive, severe disease and mortality for COVID-19 in South Asian and Black individuals, compared to White individuals, would be eliminated *if high levels of deprivation were reduced* within the population. They concluded that:

> [I]nterventions aimed at reducing material deprivation within the whole population could act to substantially reduce ethnic inequalities in the risk of COVID-19 outcomes. Specifically, a hypothetical intervention to move the 25% most deprived out of material deprivation would eliminate 40–50% of the relative excess risk for developing COVID-19 outcomes in SAB [South Asian and Black] compared to White populations. A more extreme intervention to move the 50% most deprived out of material deprivation would eliminate over 80% of the excess risk. These findings suggest the central importance of material deprivation in driving ethnic inequalities for COVID-19 outcomes. (Razieh et al, 2021: 642)

Social distancing measures also meant that many older people spent more time in unsafe and hazardous homes. Ten million people are living in 'non-decent homes' in England, two million of whom are aged 55 and over

(Centre for Ageing Better, 2020). Non-decent homes are defined as being in a state of disrepair and/or having insufficiently modern facilities. Those who are more likely to live in poor housing are often the same groups who are vulnerable to COVID-19. The Centre for Ageing Better (2020) report 'Homes, health and COVID-19' highlights the extent to which the pandemic has amplified housing–related health inequalities in the UK: first, through the acceleration of the virus in areas of poor housing; and, second, through measures to control the virus which have deepened health inequalities for those restricted to their homes. Ethnic minority groups have been among the worst affected by the deterioration of the housing stock. Data from the English Household Survey found that only 2 per cent of White British households experienced overcrowding, compared with 24 per cent of Bangladeshi households, 18 per cent of Pakistani households and 16 per cent of Black African households (gov.uk, 2020). Given this context, shielding and self-isolation posed particular problems for older people from ethnic minority groups, with the accompanying danger of risk of exposure to infection from COVID-19.

Sze et al (2020) argue that within a health-care context, the experience of discrimination and marginalisation

> contributes to inequities in the delivery of care, barriers to accessing care, loss of trust, and psycho-social stressors. There is evidence to suggest that ethnic minorities and migrant groups have been less likely to implement public health measures, be tested, or seek care when experiencing symptoms due to such barriers and inequities in the availability and accessibility of care, underscoring critical health disparities. (Sze et al, 2020: 12)

Research focusing specifically on the experiences of ethnic minority older people during the pandemic has been relatively sparse, resulting in a lack of evidence to formulate adequate policy solutions for this important group (Hewitt and Kapadia, 2021; Watkinson et al, 2021). The large-scale survey of the social consequences of COVID-19 reported by Fancourt et al found '42 per cent of people from ethnic minority backgrounds reported that they had experienced discrimination for a variety of factors in the first few months of the pandemic, whereas among white people, only 24 per cent had suffered discrimination' (2022: 34). However, aggregating the experiences of ethnic minority groups through the label Black, Asian and Minority Ethnic (BAME) 'obscures the important differences in experiences and health outcomes for these groups during the pandemic' (British Academy, 2021: 20). Recognising heterogeneity between groups is important for understanding the complexities of ethnic inequalities in health, with differences between some ethnic minority groups greater than those between any given ethnic minority group and the White British ethnic group (Watkinson et al, 2021).

Living in areas of multiple deprivation

For older populations, research indicates that the pandemic exposed 'longstanding mechanisms of exclusion and entrenched, multiple forms of disadvantage' (Walsh et al, 2021: 18), with an over-representation in deaths from COVID-19 of older adults living in areas of multiple deprivation. Watkinson et al argue that: 'Area-level social deprivation and individual socioeconomic status are important determinants of health, and intersect with gender, ethnic group, and other personal characteristics, such as immigrant status or religion, resulting in complex moderation or exacerbation of disadvantage among different groups' (Watkinson et al, 2021: 153).

Research reviewed by Buffel et al (2021) suggests that older people living in socio-economically deprived urban areas are particularly disadvantaged in times of crises, especially those associated with climate change. But the COVID-19 pandemic has added a further dimension. In particular, older people who were required to shield or follow social distancing guidelines experienced 'a double lockdown' – suffering the effects of enforced social isolation (as a result of instructions to self-isolate) while living in places which had experienced the loss of services and social infrastructure over the decade leading up to the pandemic (Marmot et al, 2020).

Research based on the English Longitudinal Study of Ageing, carried out just before the pandemic hit, demonstrated a causal relationship between area deprivation and social exclusion in later life (Prattley et al, 2020). The study revealed that older people living in deprived urban neighbourhoods had the highest levels of social exclusion compared with more affluent neighbourhoods, with evidence pointing to barriers experienced across a range of domains of exclusion, including access to services and amenities, social relationships, and civic, cultural and leisure participation. As a result, many older people living in deprived neighbourhoods may be at risk of being isolated from the social networks of support and social connections that are essential to maintaining a sense of well-being and belonging (Lewis, 2018; Yarker, 2020).

Deaths from COVID-19 for all social groups have been unevenly distributed across regions and communities. Research by Kontopantelis et al (2022), quantifying years of life lost as a result of the pandemic, found the greatest impact on the most deprived areas of England and Wales. Between March and December 2020, 1,645 years of life were lost per 100,000 of the population in the most deprived areas, compared with 916 years in the most affluent (see also Munford et al, 2022). The figures illustrate that almost twice as many years of life were lost in the very poorest areas of the country compared with the wealthiest. In the case of GM, the region which formed the context for the research discussed in this book, more than a quarter of deaths, in the first wave of the pandemic, were among people living in the most deprived communities of the region (Greater Manchester Independent Inequalities Commission, 2021).

The negative effects of social distancing on older people's physical and mental health (Bailey et al, 2021) have been further exacerbated by a lack of access to sources of social support linked to structural disadvantage, neighbourhood deprivation and cuts to local services. Disinvestment in social infrastructure in the UK has resulted in the closure of libraries, day-care centres and social clubs. Such resources are essential for providing informal spaces for people to meet, and both support and empower vulnerable groups. Deep cuts to local authorities in the decade preceding the pandemic have resulted in significant financial pressures on all public services. Cuts to funding from central government have led to a 17 per cent fall in councils' spending on local public services since 2009–2010 – equal to 23 per cent or nearly £300 per person (Institute for Fiscal Studies, 2019), which left them poorly prepared for coping with a crisis on the scale of the pandemic. COVID-19 has 'exacerbated existing structural and social inequality, with particularly negative health outcomes for those already disadvantaged in society' (British Academy, 2021: 7). In sum, the pandemic has reinforced existing inequalities in ageing along the lines of gender, class, ethnicity, race, ability and sexuality (Buffel et al, 2021).

Neighbourhoods and the organisations and groups within them are an important source of support and everyday contact for older people. However, they were also impacted by a number of trends affecting the organisation of community life coming into the pandemic. The British Academy (2021), in their review of the changing nature of communities, highlighted four main developments: first, a slow decline in people's sense of neighbourhood belonging; second, a shift to people finding a sense of community in virtual spaces and online; third, the effects of austerity policies on social and community resilience, affecting services such as public health; and, fourth, loss of funding to support essential social infrastructure (see further, Yarker, 2022a). As a result of these factors, many older people living in deprived neighbourhoods were at increased risk of being isolated from the social connections essential to maintain a sense of well-being and belonging (Lewis, 2018; Yarker, 2022a). Marmot et al (2020), for example, traced changes in health inequalities over the period 2010–2020 in England, documenting the rise in deprivation affecting many parts of the country. The authors highlighted the problems facing what the researchers termed 'left behind' and 'ignored communities' experiencing the effects of long-term deprivation:

> Over the last 10 years, these ... communities and areas have seen vital physical and community assets lost, resources and funding reduced,

community and voluntary sector services decimated and public services cut, all of which have damaged health and widened inequalities. These lost assets and services compound the multiple economic and social deprivations, including high rates of persistent poverty and low income, high levels of debt, poor health and poor housing that are already faced by many residents. (Marmot et al, 2020: 94)

The evidence suggests, therefore, that particular groups and communities were always going to be vulnerable to the threat posed by COVID-19. The more 'precarious' environment to which they were exposed made this much more likely. In the final section of this chapter, we review the meaning of precarity and its implications for understanding the social impact of COVID-19.

Living with precarity

The argument so far in this chapter is that the impact of COVID-19 was vastly increased by pre-existing social inequalities experienced by older people, ethnic minority groups and people living in areas of multiple deprivation. We have also argued that the dominant model of care and support to older people within the health-care system – defined as biomedicalisation – became highly problematic in its consequences for older people at various points of the pandemic – notably in their treatment in residential and nursing homes but also in the wider proliferation of ageist attitudes affecting cultural and social institutions. These trends have also to be located within processes which are leading to various forms of risk and vulnerability, or the impact of living in a more 'precarious world' (Grenier et al, 2020).

Farrar suggests that global trends are aligning to cause more frequent and complex epidemics: 'Climate and ecological change, urbanisation, changes in food production and habitat loss are re-shaping the way we interact with animals, boosting the chances of new diseases' (Farrar, 2021: 212). Horton (2021) cites the work of Ulrich Beck (1986) whose book *The Risk Society* explored how the creation of wealth in modern societies was always accompanied by the production of new risks, with the emergence of new viruses as one such example. Such risks are especially dangerous to groups such as older populations (and particular groups within the older population), for whom environments of inequality and austerity increase levels of exposure to the impact of the pandemic (Bambra et al, 2021). But a further dimension to understanding the impact of the virus is to locate it within the context of the emergence of a precarious world, characterised by insecure forms of labour (Standing, 2011), privatised health and social care (Simmonds, 2021), and intense forms of discrimination facing ethnic minority groups, people with a disability and those from the LGBTQ+ community.

Although some variations exist in its associated meanings, 'precarity' is used most often to refer to the insecurities, unwanted risks and hazards of contemporary life, typically associated with globalisation and neoliberal economic and social policies. One of the most widely cited references to precarity, and more specifically precariousness, is that of Butler who views it as a 'politically induced condition in which certain populations suffer from failing social and economic networks of support and become differentially exposed to injury, violence and death' (Butler, 2009: 25). This 'differential' exposure was especially acute for older people in the context of COVID-19 because of the interaction between their medical conditions (for example, multiple morbidities), and the social context, with the impact of austerity in reducing levels of support for vulnerable populations (Simmonds, 2021). The broader point is that pre-existing conditions – various forms of economic and social precarity – contributed significantly to elevating the risk of infection for groups such as older people, contributing to the severity of their impact and the likelihood of their eventual death. These pre-existing conditions also left older people exposed to ageism and inequalities in treatment both in health and social care settings, as evidenced earlier in this chapter.

Precarity offers a lens to understand new and sustained forms of insecurity affecting later life associated with economic pressures on public services, unstable forms of employment and negative perceptions about population ageing (Grenier et al, 2020). The concept helps to shed light on the politics of ageing, whereby older people may suffer from unequal access to material goods and diminished social networks. Precarity can become particularly acute in later life, as a result of the accumulation of disadvantage in the context of contemporary social, economic and political conditions (Dannefer, 2021). Portacolone et al point to specific markers of precarity, which are likely to be especially relevant to older adults living alone, including managing 'compounding pressures' such as limited access to appropriate services and retaining independence (Portacolone et al, 2021: 251).

The concept of precarity further emphasises the *interdependence of lives* across the life-course. It suggests that intimate social relationships, especially those relating to family and friendship, are often where precarity is felt, as well-being is inextricably dependent on the choices, behaviours and resources of others. As Settersten argues: 'Who we become, the opportunities we are given or denied, the decisions we make, the actions we take, the meanings we derive—these are all intimately tangled up in social relationships' (Settersten, 2015: 217). From a life-course perspective, precarity can occur in multiple life domains, such as family, employment or education. Settersten suggests that: 'Precarity in one domain can interact with and spill over into others. So, too, can precarity in one domain be reduced or offset by the strength of stability in other domains' (Settersten, 2020: 21).

This approach is especially relevant for understanding how people manage public health crises such as COVID-19, in order to examine both their immediate circumstances as well as transitions and events experienced through the life-course. Our study plays particular attention to how social relationships were changed in the context of COVID-19, and in a wider environment of insecurity and risk facing people living in lower-income communities.

Conclusion

The argument of this book is that the pandemic should be understood within the broader context of ageing itself becoming a more *precarious experience*, with (in the UK) reductions in social protection, the raising of pension ages, the privatisation of health and social care, and the impact of various forms of discrimination facing groups from ethnic minority communities (Simmonds, 2021). This environment is important in influencing how people reacted to and managed the pandemic, and in particular the resources which they had at their disposal. Precarity is produced by unequal social arrangements, which can become particularly acute in later life, as a result of the accumulation of disadvantage and the contemporary social, economic and political context (Grenier et al, 2020).

But the question we explore in this book is how – faced with a pandemic playing through lives already affected by deep-rooted inequalities of various kinds – people, and the communities in which they lived, managed and organised their everyday lives. *What kinds of responses did they have to the imposition of lockdowns and social distancing? How did their daily routines change? How did these interact with the inequalities affecting their lives? How did community organisations, working in areas with high levels of deprivation, respond in providing help and support?* These were some of the questions that were examined by talking to older people and the community organisations which support them over the course of 2020 and 2021. Before reviewing our findings, we first discuss the methodology developed for our research.

3

Methodology of the study

Introduction

This chapter outlines the *research methodology* and reflects on the different stages of the research process. The overall aim of the study was to examine the impact of social distancing measures on everyday life, as well as to contribute evidence to assist local, regional and national organisations working on behalf of older people. The pandemic raised challenges for social research, both because of the impact and abruptness of the initial lockdown in March 2020, and its variable consequences for different groups within the older population. At the same time, the pandemic also offered new possibilities for undertaking research, given the need to create alternatives to conventional styles of fieldwork (Tarrant et al, 2021).

The chapter is divided into five main parts: first, the *qualitative, longitudinal design* of the study is described, along with details about the collaborative relationships developed with partner organisations involved in the study. Second, the process of *working with community organisations* and recruiting participants is discussed. Third, a description of the *data collection process* follows, explaining how telephone interviews were conducted both with community organisations and older people themselves. Fourth, we explain how we carried out the *data analysis* which included thematic and longitudinal approaches. Lastly, we provide some context about the geographical area – *Greater Manchester* – in which the research was conducted.

Methodological approach

The research followed a qualitative longitudinal approach in order to explore the impact of the pandemic in the 12 months from March 2020. Longitudinal qualitative research can be distinguished from other qualitative approaches by the way in which time is embedded in the research process, making *change* in people's lives a key focus for analysis (Emmel and Hughes, 2010). Following Settersten and colleagues, we took the view that qualitative longitudinal research was

> best suited for uncovering the breadth and diversity of individual situations and subjective responses to the threat of illness and public health restrictions meant to contain it. For example, individual interpretations of experiences of quarantine, alterations to their sense

of control, and efforts to exercise agency and maintain a sense of well-being in the face of the pandemic are varied and nuanced and not well-assessed by fixed-choice survey questions. (Settersten et al, 2020: 9)

The longitudinal design enabled us to explore older people's lives as heterogeneous and dynamic, amidst evolving socio-cultural and socio-historical circumstances (Lekkas et al, 2017). Interviewing the same individuals at different time points, our aim was to examine older people's lived experiences, against the backdrop of (in this case) the lockdowns imposed because of COVID-19, and changes affecting individuals' immediate familial and social environments.

The project team drew upon an extensive network of organisations from the voluntary sector in GM, including those working in particular neighbourhoods, or with specific minority communities of identity or experiences. We also liaised regularly with statutory services and local authorities across the region. The Greater Manchester Combined Authority Ageing Hub provided extensive help and support throughout the project and also introduced the project team to some of the organisations with whom the project worked. The Ageing Hub co-ordinates Age-Friendly work in GM and brings together universities in the region, the voluntary sector, public and not-for-profit organisations, and the people who live and work across GM, to improve the lives of residents as they age.

A growing body of research, to which members of the research team have contributed, emphasises the importance of using *collaborative or co-research approaches* to ensure that the lives of under-represented groups are represented fairly and accurately (see, for example, Lewis and Cotterell, 2018; Yarker and Buffel, 2022). Where possible, our research followed a participatory ethos, following principles of openness, flexibility, sensitivity and responsiveness (Littlechild et al, 2015). The project team greatly benefited from working with networks with whom they already had prior relationships, with a Research Advisory Board established representing various organisations who supported the study. The Board included representatives from the Manchester Ethnic Health Forum, the Greater Manchester Combined Authority Ageing Hub, Age-Friendly Manchester and the Centre for Policy on Ageing. These organisations provided advice and feedback on the development of the research design, sampling strategies and dissemination. Working closely with the Board was vital for the study, due to our focus on marginalised groups experiencing exclusion, stigma and discrimination (see also Fenge et al, 2010). The study was approved by the University of Manchester School of Social Sciences Ethics Committee.

The sample

Interviews with community organisations

The first stage of the research comprised interviews with a range of organisations, including statutory service providers, community and voluntary sector centres, neighbourhood associations, and local government initiatives supporting older people. While not all organisations focused solely on the needs of older populations, all ran activities and services which catered for people aged 50 and over. The 21 participating organisations (see Table 3.1) acted as gatekeepers for this research. Community organisers were asked to provide names of older people who might be willing to be interviewed, with particular reference to those at risk of some form of social exclusion.

Representatives from the organisations were also asked to share their insights through interviews on, in the majority of cases, two separate occasions from March 2020 to February 2021. In a number of cases, members of the project team had more frequent contact with the organisations throughout the period of the study. The interviews included questions such as: *What have been the main changes to your organisation and role? What kinds of support were you able to offer people during the pandemic? What are the challenges your organisation faces? What are the main lessons learned from the last 12 months?*

Since the restrictions brought about by the COVID-19 lockdown rules were unprecedented, the research team had to quickly devise alternative ways of working, largely using online platforms. From March 2020, face-to-face meetings were prohibited, meaning that all interactions with community organisations and older people were carried out by email, video-call or telephone. The researchers were concerned about the potential of the project to place *extra pressure on community and voluntary sector groups* who were already working at capacity, adapting their services rapidly to deliver support to older people, such as emergency food deliveries (see Chapter 8). To try and avoid this, correspondence was kept to a minimum and meetings were organised flexibly to fit around the organisations' changing demands.

Interviews with older people

The second stage of the research involved telephone interviews with 102 older people from a variety of backgrounds. A purposive sample was recruited through the community organisations, based on the following criteria: age, gender, ethnicity and sexual orientation. The sample was drawn from those 50 and over in order to capture experiences among groups where cumulative disadvantage can lead to poorer health outcomes at earlier ages, compared to more advantaged groups. Life expectancy in GM is close to two years below the England average, and healthy life expectancy three years below the England average (Marmot et al, 2020). The South Asian participants were

Table 3.1: List of organisations

Name	Type of organisation
Age-Friendly Manchester	A partnership involving organisations, groups and individuals across the city playing their part in making Manchester a great place to grow older.
Age-Friendly Manchester Older People's Board	The Board includes and represents older people, addressing issues affecting the quality of life for older residents and their communities across Manchester.
Age UK Salford	An independent charity working in Salford to offer support and direct services to older people.
Age UK Wigan	An independent charity working in the Borough of Wigan to offer support and services to older people.
Ambition for Ageing	A £10.2 million programme that aimed to create more age-friendly places in GM and empower people to live fulfilling lives as they age.
Brunswick Church	Inner-city community church.
Brunswick Estate Men's Group	A community group for men living on an inner-city estate at risk of social isolation.
Caribbean and African Health Network	A network established to eradicate health inequalities within a generation for Caribbean and African people.
Collyhurst Lalley Centre	A community centre, food pantry and community allotment based in North Manchester.
Ethnic Health Forum	A non-profit, charitable organisation registered with Charity Commission, England.
Greater Manchester Ageing Hub	The Greater Manchester Combined Authority's strategic response to opportunities and challenges of an ageing population in GM.
Greater Manchester Older People's Network	A network of people aged 50 and above and organisational representatives working for positive change for older people in GM.
Hopton Hopefuls Tenants Group	A group of tenants who organise together to improve life for older tenants at Hopton Court in Hulme and also run a weekly savings club.
Inspiring Communities Together	A Charitable Incorporated Organisation which helps older people feel more connected with their community in Salford.
Kashmiri Youth Project	An independent charity dedicated to the development and economic regeneration of the communities of Rochdale.
Levenshulme Good Neighbours	A registered charity that works to offer practical, social and emotional support to older people living in Levenshulme.
Levenshulme Inspire	A social enterprise offering community-led services that promote the well-being of residents of Levenshulme and beyond.
LGBT Foundation	A national charity delivering advice, support and information services to LGBT communities.

(continued)

Table 3.1: List of organisations (continued)

Name	Type of organisation
Manchester BME Network	The network strives to support Black and minority ethnic groups and organisations of all sizes to become more effective and successful and to play their full part in contributing to communities in Manchester.
NHS Public Health and Community Engagement	Place-based groups that co-ordinated COVID-19 responses among other duties.
Tameside Grafton Community Centre	A community hub catering for local residents offering a range of weekly activities to suit everyone.

recruited through the Kashmiri Youth Project (KYP) based in Rochdale, the Ethnic Health Forum based in Rusholme and the Manchester BAME Network working across Manchester. The African Caribbean participants were recruited through the Caribbean and African Health Network, and the LGBTQ+ participants were recruited through the LGBT foundation. The remaining White British participants were recruited through the other community organisations.

Participants came from 30 neighbourhoods across GM (see Figure 3.1), including: Levenshulme, Tameside, Salford, Wigan, Brunswick, Hulme, Middleton, Rochdale, Bury, Stockport, Moss Side, Trafford, Chorlton, Cheetham Hill, Crumpsall, Heaton Chapel, Bolton, Worsley, Northern Quarter, Ancoats, Sale, Wilmslow, Fallowfield, Charleston, Openshaw, Stretford, Whalley Range, Rusholme, Wythenshawe and Northern Moor.

In order to minimise withdrawals from the study, the same researcher carried out the repeat interviews, with the aim of building trust and rapport through the duration of the research. From the sample of 102 interviewed, 99 agreed to take part in a second interview and 88 agreed to take part in a third. Reasons for not participating in the second interview included: travelling abroad to visit family (1); poor health (1); and not interested in being interviewed (1). In the third interview, reasons for not participating included: poor health (4); return to country of origin (4); not interested in being interviewed (2), and four were unable to be contacted. All of the quotations in this book include a pseudonym to protect the anonymity of participants, as well as their age and how they describe their identity.

Data collection

Interviewing during COVID-19 produced both challenges and opportunities. For example, social distancing restrictions meant that all interviews had to be conducted over the telephone, and face-to-face interactions with participants, which are valuable for developing rapport (such as eye contact and smiling)

Figure 3.1: Map of Greater Manchester

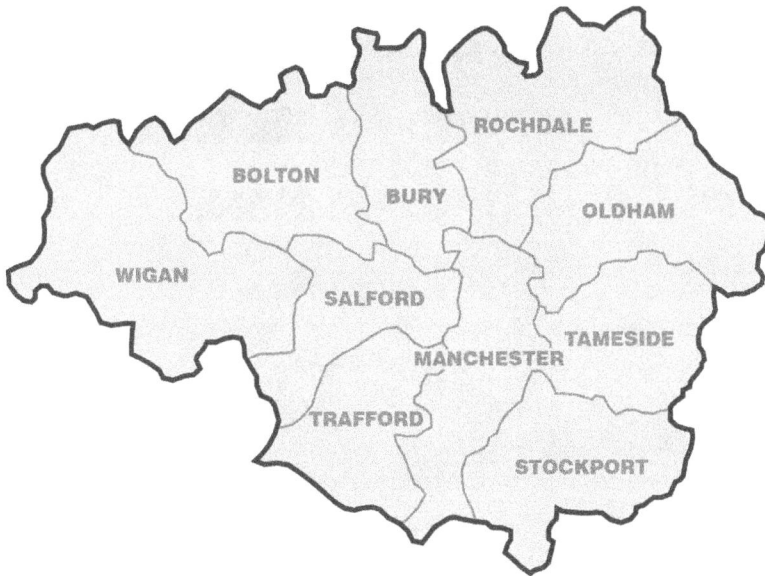

Table 3.2: Interviews with older people

Interview number	Date	Number of interviews
First interview	May–August 2020	102
Second interview	June–November 2020	99
Third interview	January–February 2021	88

were not possible. In other circumstances, the interviews with older people would have been carried out in person. On the telephone, the research team were unable to capture the unspoken elements of conversations, such as hand gestures and body language, which are important dimensions of interviews. Also, many of the interviewees discussed stressful events affecting their lives and the researchers were mindful about the limitations of using telephone interviews for exploring sensitive issues (see also Bundy et al, 2021). In this context, participants were given the opportunity to have a break, or for the interview to be arranged for another occasion.

Although limited in some regards, carrying out interviews by telephone made the data-collection process efficient and relatively inexpensive (Sturges and Hanrahan, 2004). Multiple interviews could be carried out in one day, as the researchers did not have to spend time travelling between interviews. Further, in some cases, telephone interviews may have allowed respondents to disclose sensitive information more freely (Novick, 2008), due to the

Figure 3.2: Age and gender of participants

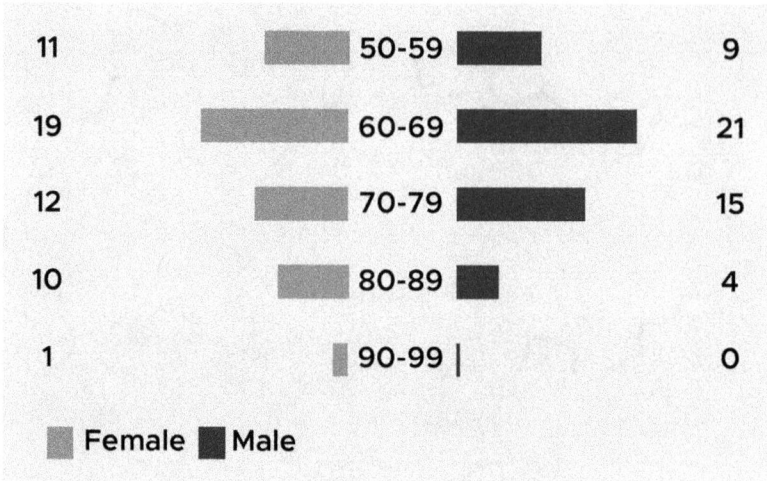

11	50-59	9
19	60-69	21
12	70-79	15
10	80-89	4
1	90-99	0

■ Female ■ Male

Figure 3.3: Ethnic background of participants

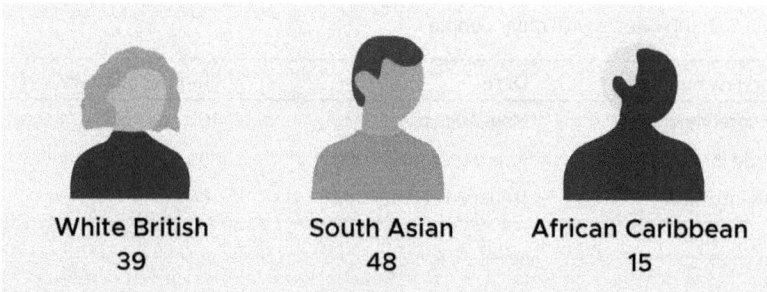

White British	South Asian	African Caribbean
39	48	15

anonymity of talking to a researcher remotely (Tarrant et al, 2021). Another benefit of carrying out telephone interviews was that the researcher could offer flexibility for participants, providing them with control over the time and spaces where the interview took place (Irvine et al, 2013). The interviews were conducted 'in situ' (May and Lewis, 2020), as most of our participants were spending the majority of their time in their dwelling, and therefore a lot of the conversation centred on the home, surrounding environment, family and everyday lives. Because the interviews were carried out on the telephone from home, some participants reflected that they felt more at ease and comfortable being in a familiar environment, as one participant explained: "I don't think I'd talk as much if I was face to face with anybody."

The telephone interviews also offered some participants with an activity to do during the periods of lockdown, and an opportunity to talk at length

Figure 3.4: Housing tenure of participants

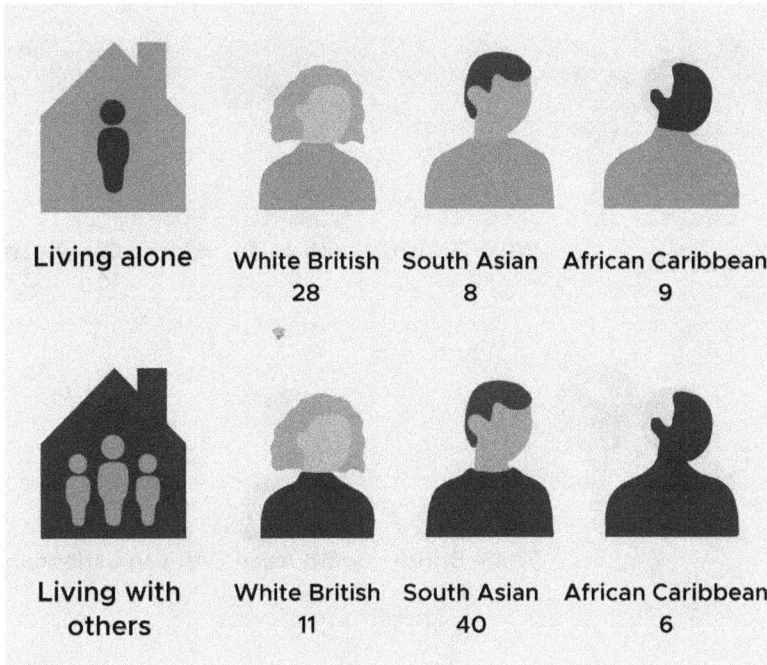

| Living alone | White British 28 | South Asian 8 | African Caribbean 9 |

| Living with others | White British 11 | South Asian 40 | African Caribbean 6 |

when opportunities to socialise were limited. Some participants told us that they looked forward to their interview, as the appointment with the researcher gave some structure to their day. Others noted how the questions made them reflect on the pandemic and think about their everyday lives in a different way. One participant described the interviews as cathartic, explaining: "[W]hen you ring me, I don't know what I'm going to say, but when I start talking it just kind of flows; it's been quite healthy." However, in other cases, participants were reluctant to talk at length, as they were suffering from a health problem, or coming to terms with bereavement, or just felt "fed up".

The interviews were semi-structured, allowing the participants to guide the discussion, and to have plenty of time to talk about topics which were important to their own situation. This approach was adopted to allow participants to discuss their experiences at length, and in their own words (Whitehead and Torossian, 2021). Before the repeat interviews, the researcher read through the previous transcript(s) and made notes on specific themes which arose, so they could tailor the questions according to each participant. The aim was to pick up on issues or subjects addressed in each interview, and to try and make the exchanges like a conversation which continued over time. For the second and third interviews, the research team developed a different

Figure 3.5: Household composition of participants

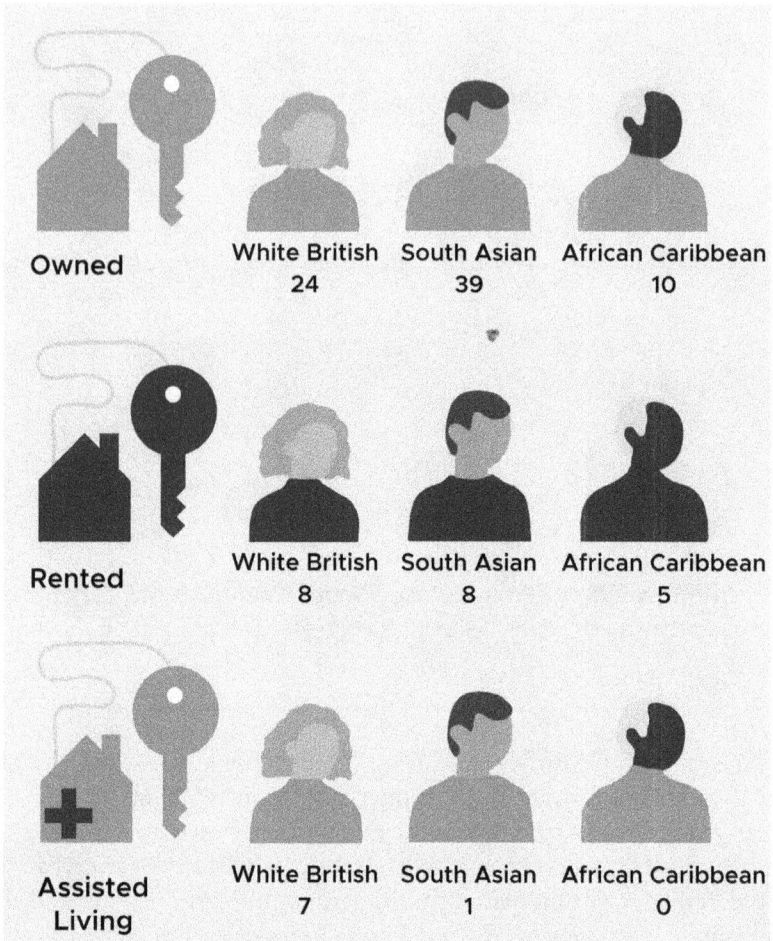

	White British	South Asian	African Caribbean
Owned	24	39	10
Rented	8	8	5
Assisted Living	7	1	0

set of interview questions to build on the findings from each interview. Overall, the majority of the interviews provoked richly detailed discussions.

The interviews with community members were carried out by the project team, with the exception of participants from the South Asian community. Informed consent was requested over the telephone at the beginning of each interview. The interviews were recorded and transcribed, with each one lasting for an average of 50 minutes. The interviews included questions such as:

- How has *everyday life* changed since social distancing rules were introduced?
- What does an *average day* consist of?
- How have *relationships* changed with family, friends and neighbours?

Figure 3.6: Number of children of participants

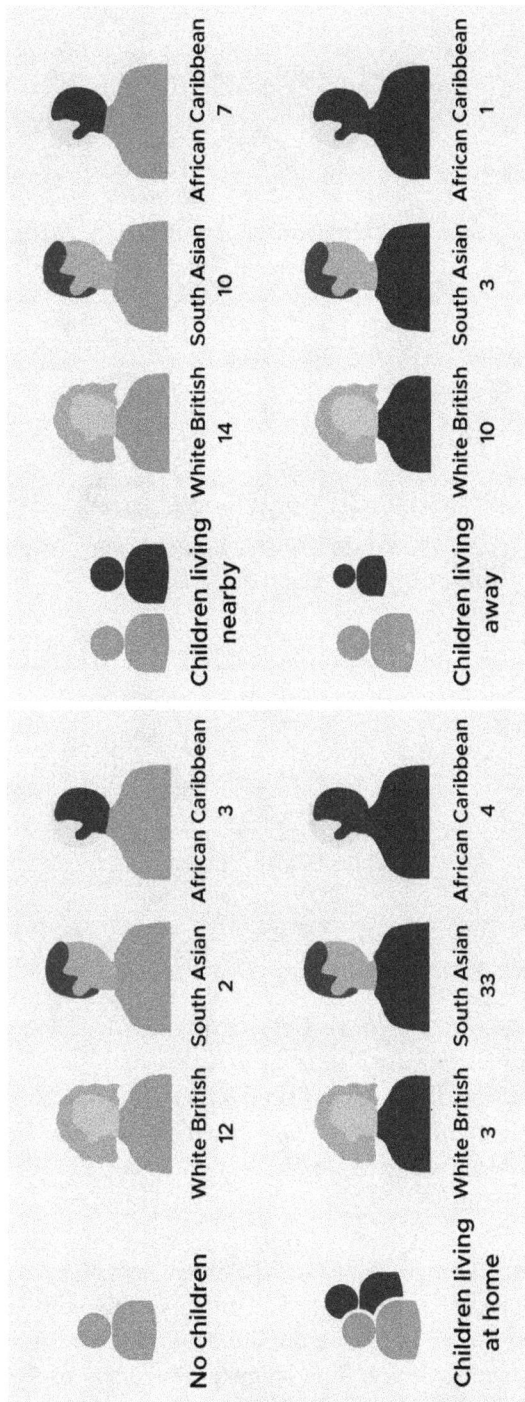

Figure 3.7: Self-ascribed health of participants

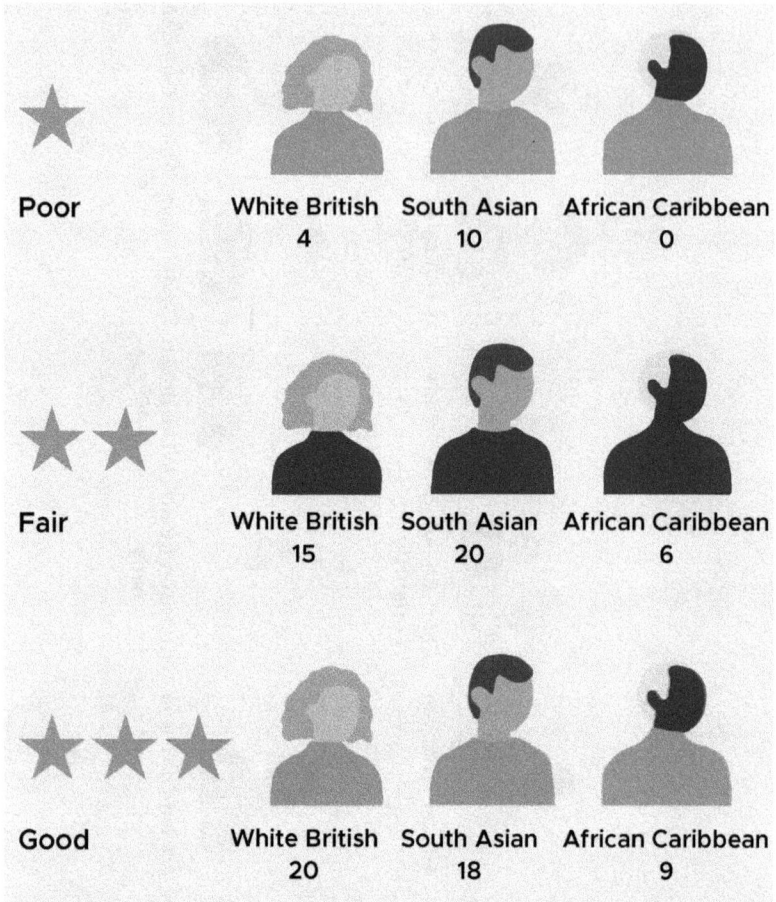

★

Poor

White British	South Asian	African Caribbean
4	10	0

★★

Fair

White British	South Asian	African Caribbean
15	20	6

★★★

Good

White British	South Asian	African Caribbean
20	18	9

- How have older people been using *online* or equivalent forms of communication?
- How has social distancing affected *mental and physical health*?
- Can people identify areas of *support* which would be helpful to them?
- What *resources* do people draw on to cope with lockdown and social distancing?

For the South Asian participants, the interviews were conducted by staff and volunteers from the respective organisations who understood some of the cultural sensitivities surrounding the research, and in the language of the participants' choice. The languages used to conduct the interviews included Urdu, Hindi, Punjabi, Pahari, Swahili and English, with a combination of more than one language in some cases. The interview schedule was shared with the organisation in advance and a briefing with the lead representatives of the organisation was held with the project team. This gave the organisation a chance to offer any feedback on the interview schedule, particularly around whether or not any of the questions might be culturally insensitive, inappropriate or should be phrased differently. At the request of the organisations, these interviews were not audio-recorded but detailed notes were taken and translated into English where necessary.

By collaborating with organisations who work with South Asian communities, the research team were able to recruit members of the older population from a variety of backgrounds. However, such collaborations are not without challenges and there are important aspects to reflect upon in relation to how they shaped the data collection. First, these interviews were carried out by staff and volunteers at the organisations because they were able to communicate with the participants in their chosen language and dialect and because they were closer to the participants in terms of their cultural and religious backgrounds. In many cases, the interviewers already knew the participants, which meant that it was often easier for them to develop a rapport between them which is essential in making the person being interviewed feel more comfortable (Clough et al, 2006).

The 'closeness' between the interviewers and interviewees also presented challenges. For example, when comparing participants' transcripts across the three interviews there were some discrepancies in the participant's age. After further discussion with the community organisations, it became apparent that some of the younger interviewers were reluctant to ask the participant's age directly due to cultural norms that made this inappropriate. Some interviewees estimated the age of the participant and because each participant was not interviewed by the same person inconsistencies occurred in the information collected about each participant. There were also variations between the interview responses, in relation to the quality and depth of the data due to different staff and volunteers carrying out the interviews. Interviewers for the South Asian sample were chosen based on the language and dialect they spoke, and some had less experience of interviewing than others.

Data analysis

All interviews were coded and analysed by one of the researchers using NVivo, a computer software program designed to facilitate content and thematic analysis, and verified by the other members of the project team who analysed sub-samples of the data and compared results to check for consistency. The coding was carried out according to themes identified in the secondary literature (see Chapter 2), as well as those which emerged in the interview transcripts, both of which were incorporated into the coding framework. They included: experiences of social distancing; impact of COVID-19 on physical and mental health; and relationships with friends and family. Parts of the transcripts that were relevant according to each theme were selected. Regular virtual meetings were held to discuss ongoing coding and exchange insights as well as to rectify inconsistencies in how the coding framework was being interpreted.

A *cross-sectional* analysis was then conducted, to look at how themes emerged across the whole dataset. The interviews were analysed according to themes which helped to identify recurring patterns across the interviews (for example, people's common experiences of social distancing; the impact of digital exclusion; deterioration in physical and mental health) and previously unexpected trends (for example, the role of religion among participants' everyday lives). The analysis enabled the research team to verify how often certain words and phrases were used by participants (for example, words such as 'lonely', 'depressed' or 'prayer'), and to compare responses between different groups within the sample (for example, how many times people talked about gardening activities or exercising outdoors). The data was then analysed *longitudinally*, examining how responses changed (or stayed the same) over time from one interview to the next, for each participant.

Case study: Greater Manchester

This section provides some context on GM, the case study in this research. GM comprises ten local authorities and is the country's second most populous urban area, with almost three million people living in the city-region. GM has had a 6.9 per cent increase in its population over the past ten years according to the 2021 Census (compared with a 6.3 per cent growth for England and Wales). Some of the local authorities within GM include some of the most *culturally diverse* areas in the UK with a long history of migration from different parts of the world. During the Industrial Revolution, the area was the heart of intense urban growth and attracted migrants from a range of backgrounds, including Pakistani, Indian, Chinese, African and African Caribbean communities. From the early 2000s, many skilled workers from Europe, India and West Africa were also attracted by employment opportunities in Manchester – as information technology (IT) professionals, for example, helping transform the city into a tech hub for the north of England. Many were also drawn to work in the health and care sector, with nurses coming from countries outside the EU making a vital contribution to the NHS (Sassen and Arun, 2017). Manchester is the only city outside London to have residents in each of the 90 listed ethnic groups in the census, and has over 200 languages spoken. Results from the 2021 census show a 40 per cent increase in the population from a BAME background since 2011 (Manchester City Council, 2022).

As well as being characterised by population change, GM has also been reshaped by *deindustrialisation*. Between the 1960s and the early 1990s, GM experienced a dramatic loss of industries, as the outsourcing of mass production went to countries in the Global South (Lewis and Symons, 2018). Since that time, ambitious regeneration projects have been established across the city-region, aimed at transforming some of the most deprived neighbourhoods. Urban redevelopment has also prompted significant population growth, especially at the centre of the conurbation in Manchester (ONS, 2022d).

Demographic trends for GM indicate growth in the numbers of people 75 and over living alone (from 97,000 in 2011 to a projected 161,000 in 2036). It is expected that 14 per cent of the GM population will be 75 and over by 2036, a group identified at particular risk of social exclusion and social isolation (GMCA, 2017). Life expectancy – and healthy life expectancy – in some parts of Greater Manchester are amongst the lowest in the UK. Men and women aged 65 years in Manchester have the lowest life expectancy compared to other areas of the UK – men 15.9 years; women 18.8 years. This compares to 21.6 years for men in Kensington and Chelsea and 24.6 years for women in Camden. By 2035, almost one in three GM residents aged 65 or over are likely to have a limiting long-term illness that affects their day-to-day activities in some way. COVID-19 has taken a significant toll on the physical and mental health of older people across GM, increased in many instances by the challenges they were already facing before the pandemic.

The Greater Manchester Independent Inequalities Commission (2021) describes how even before the pandemic, the region was 'fractured by inequalities' across a range of indicators. Significant concentrations of income deprivation can be found across the city-region. Almost half of GM areas are within the 30 per cent most income-deprived areas in England. Some 80,540 pensioners in GM claim pension credits, reflecting cumulative inequality arising from low incomes, long-term unemployment and poor health (ONS, 2019). Healthy life expectancy at birth ends as early as age 60 for both men and women in GM (GMCA, 2018). A GM-based study, examining the benefits of urban green infrastructure on older people, found that, with the exception of public parks and other green areas, all other types of urban green and blue space (for example, canals) were smaller on average compared with the most affluent neighbourhoods (Lindley et al, 2020). The authors found that:

> In some neighbourhoods with older residents on lower incomes there [was] very little green and blue space at all. ... Some older people ... have far fewer opportunities to receive urban green infrastructure related benefits and fewer opportunities to contribute to protecting, maintaining and enhancing local urban and green and blue spaces. This can be a source of health inequalities. (Lindley et al, 2020)

In the first wave of the pandemic in 2020, more than a quarter of deaths in GM were among people living in the most deprived areas of the region (Greater Manchester Independent Inequalities Commission, 2018). The higher COVID-19 infection and death rates experienced by people of Bangladeshi, Pakistani and Black ethnicity can in large part be explained by their concentration in more densely populated, deprived areas, characterised by multiple types of inequality. This context suggests that social exclusion is likely to have increased during the period of the pandemic, with the worst effects being found among those already affected by long-term inequalities of various kinds. Digital exclusion is especially relevant in the context of GM, where Office for National Statistics data from 2019 revealed that 57 per cent of people aged 75 and over had not used the internet in the past three months or had never used the internet (ONS, 2021). Ayalon et al (2021) note that digital exclusion may be especially risky for some older adults, preventing them from accessing goods and services and obtaining the social support they may require during the pandemic.

Since the mid-2000s, the need to create 'age-friendly cities and communities' has emerged as a major concern for urban policy development. The World Health Organization has driven the age-friendly agenda through the development of the Global Network of Age-friendly Cities and Communities. Manchester was the first city in the UK to join the network, in 2010. The growth of the network has contributed to the development of age-friendly initiatives, addressing diverse issues such as green spaces, mobility, walkability, home adaptions and community services. Manchester has played an important role in contributing to the development of this agenda. In 2018, GM was recognised by the World Health Organization as the UK's first age-friendly city-region, celebrating the different activities under development to make the region a better place in which to grow old. The onset of COVID-19 represented a major test for the age-friendly movement, and for work in GM in particular. We return to the implications of the pandemic for age-friendly work in the penultimate chapter of this book.

Conclusion

This chapter has outlined the methodology used in the study, and explained the strategy developed to interview older people and organisations working on their behalf. The objective behind our study was to uncover the breadth and diversity of individual experiences, using a qualitative longitudinal approach. Since the restrictions brought about by the COVID-19 lockdown rules were unprecedented, the research team devised alternative ways of working, largely using online platforms and telephone interviews. An extensive network of organisations from the voluntary sector assisted the researchers to recruit a diverse group of older people to be interviewed. A purposive sample was created, to explore the experiences of people aged 50 and over from a variety of marginalised backgrounds.

The following four chapters analyse the findings from the study. Chapters 4, 5 and 6 focus on the *lived experience* of 102 older people, drawn from a variety of neighbourhoods across GM, from different social and ethnic groups. Chapter 7 then explores the interviews carried out with 21 community-based organisations (which included mutual-aid groups, voluntary bodies, neighbourhood groups and faith-based groups), examining the role these organisations played in responding to the pandemic and how their responses changed over the 12-month period.

4

Everyday life
under lockdown: relationships
and routines

Introduction

This chapter presents findings from two sets of interviews carried out from May to November 2020, together with a third interview early in 2021, exploring the impact of the pandemic and subsequent lockdowns on everyday life. The interviews discussed in this chapter highlight a number of themes: *reactions to the lockdown and changes over time; the impact of shielding; maintaining routines; shopping under lockdown; growing older under lockdown; and reflections on the impact of COVID-19*. These areas are discussed in turn, drawing upon the views and experiences reported by our participants. Chapter 5 then examines some of the themes in more depth through four case studies, and Chapter 6 focuses on issues relating to how relationships changed over the 12-month period, the provision of care under lockdown, support from neighbours, access to outdoor spaces, and the role of technology.

Experiences of lockdown

'From this evening I must give the British people a very simple instruction – you must stay at home. ... You should not be meeting friends. If your friends ask you to meet, you should say no. You should not be meeting family members who do not live in your home. You should not be going shopping except for essentials like food and medicine – and you should do as little as you can. If you don't follow the rules the police will have the powers to enforce them, including through fines and dispersing gatherings.' (Prime Minister Boris Johnson, Address to the Nation, 23 March 2020)

On 23 March 2020, the general public in the UK was ordered to stay at home, 'except for very limited purposes', including shopping for basic necessities, one form of exercise a day, and travel to work only when absolutely necessary. Some 3.8 million people were ordered to shield (almost 6 per cent of the population), 74 per cent of whom were aged 50 and over. Further, from March 2020, all those aged 70 years and over, and those deemed 'clinically vulnerable', were also advised to stay indoors and limit their interactions with others for 12 weeks. National restrictions were partially eased for a few months in the second half of 2020, but a new lockdown in England was reintroduced in November 2020 for a month, with a third starting in January 2021.

The people interviewed in our research, notably during the first lockdown, were largely supportive of the measures adopted, albeit recognising some of the challenges involved. Kamal, a 61-year-old Indian man, commented that: "Getting used to wearing a face mask isn't easy and one has to adapt. Changes are difficult to accept but for our health I have had to accept and follow the government guidelines." Azlan, a 51-year-old Pakistani man, felt that the "[g]overnment has really helped us in raising awareness about it, warning about coronavirus and that really helped me in organising my life while I'm staying home". And Joseph, a 69-year-old White British man living on his own agreed, commenting: "I think they're doing it the right way, because it's very important. They can't just, they couldn't just be foolish and release the lockdown. They've done it in stages, I agree with that."

Subsequent interviews, in the summer and autumn of 2020, found some of our participants starting to feel less confident about the rules, with concerns expressed about what seemed to be 'contradictory' messages, or a sense that measures were being eased without clear explanation. Samantha, a 69-year-old, living on her own, felt that the process had become rather arbitrary: "I don't think it's more normal, I think we have just adapted. I mean when the government began relaxing things we just knew that was idiotic, you could tell they hadn't got control of the situation." Others raised concerns about the impact of the early lifting of lockdown on the behaviour of others. Eric, a 60-year-old White British man who identified as gay, interviewed during the first lockdown, felt that: "Because things are relaxing from tomorrow, I think I'll be even more afraid of people thinking it's all over, which it isn't all over."

The impact of lockdown

Experiences of changes arising from the lockdown showed three main variations across the different groups interviewed. These were illustrated by people who experienced *no real change in their lives*; others who reported *changes to parts of their lives* which were both positive and negative; and those who felt there had been a significant *decrease* in the quality of their daily life. Unsurprisingly, the majority of our respondents (88/102) experienced a steep decline in social contacts during the period of the first lockdown, in the spring of 2020 (see also Freedman et al, 2022). The small number of participants who reported *no real change* in their contacts and activities were mainly those who considered themselves isolated to some degree prior to the onset of the pandemic. In some cases, these were people already confined to their homes, often living precarious lives associated with poor health and living on a limited income. Michael, a 64-year-old White British man living alone, reported that: "I don't really get any visitors or anything like that so nothing much has changed. I'm still just struggling along. I was depressed before and I'm still depressed now." And Rod, a 64-year-old also living alone, identified a range of personal issues:

'When you're living on your own, because [in my case] your wife has passed away ... and when you've spent the last 15 years looking after your parents through dementia and Parkinson's and cancer, all of your own local friend base drifts away. So, now that my parents have died all my friends are just no longer there and I am literally just on my own.'

The second variation refers to those who, while feeling largely positive, were still susceptible to changes of mood and negative feelings. Stewart, a 72-year-old White British man living on his own, had been an active member of a church before the lockdown. He reported being in good physical health, and in regular contact with his adult children. Yet, despite identifying many good things about his life, he also reported that social distancing had increased some of the challenges associated with living alone: "Some days I get up and I feel dreadful ... they call it a corona-coaster don't they [laughing] I think that's the new word." Other interviewees highlighted the challenges associated with spending more time at home. George, a 71-year-old White British man, living in a sheltered housing scheme where access to the communal areas had been closed off, reported: "Everyone sort of stayed in their rooms. So, I started staying in my room but after a while you are almost climbing the walls."

A third theme was expressed by participants who had felt that they had experienced a significant *decrease* in their quality of life. Sidney was a 73-year-old White British man whose wife had died some years prior to the study. He had no children but two sisters who lived some distance from Manchester. Before the pandemic, Sidney enjoyed the company of people he met at his local library and would normally have breaks away from home during the year, travelling to different places or visiting his sisters. He described:

'I was coping, my way of coping was by going to these different groups, friendship groups ... and churches, and so at least I got some sort of human contact. So ... of course ... everything stopped in March and that made me realise just how isolated I am. I didn't feel isolated before because I'd got various groups that I was going to and I can always go and sit in the local library for an hour or two if I'd got nothing else to do.'

Nikita, a 62-year-old Indian woman, also reported major social changes as a result of the lockdown. She lived alone and suffered from long-term health problems and described herself as in constant pain. She was dependent on the use of a wheelchair but was highly active before the pandemic. Nikita talked about her life during lockdown in the following way:

'My life [has] changed drastically. I would regularly see my mother, siblings and the extended family in Leicester. My daughters regularly visited me in Manchester. I also enjoyed social and leisure activities ... meeting friends for lunches, cinema, theatre, art galleries, etc. I had a routine of going to the church for art and choir, meditation practice and to the Gurdwara [Sikh temple]. ... For me ... the impact has been

Figure 4.1: Woman with mask

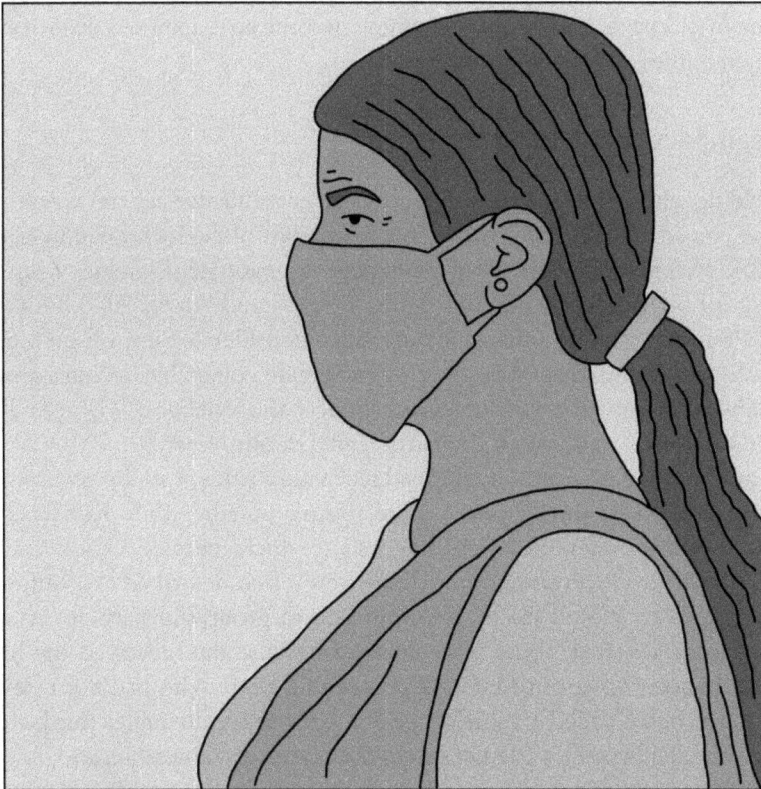

losing the human connections ... face to face and physical – hugs from my daughter, with my mother and friend.'

Douglas, who is gay, had similar feelings: "That's one thing I have felt, the kind of isolation of being a single man, 70 years old, who suddenly is cut off from all the normal social activities that he would do." Other participants reported additional pressures with the pandemic interacting with challenges in their personal lives. Paula was a 75-year-old White British woman in a same sex relationship. Her partner was undergoing treatment for cancer:

'I'm quite a busy person and the lockdown has been, for me, horrible—it's been horrible. ... The biggest change is not being able to be the social person I am ... that's the biggest change. It's a horrible change because I am and always have been for the whole of my life a social person.'

These comments illustrate how for some of our participants, ways of coping with pressures in their lives *intensified* during the first lockdown. Sidney realised 'just how isolated' he was; Douglas emphasised the challenge of being a single, older, gay man. 'Staying apart' was certainly a challenge for many of our participants, but one which in some cases exposed deep-rooted vulnerabilities and inequalities.

The impact of shielding

Shielding, either through choice or government guidance (a letter was sent to those considered clinically vulnerable at the start of the lockdown in March 2020), presented another set of challenges to negotiate. Evidence from the English Longitudinal Study of Ageing (Steptoe and Street, 2020; Di Gessa and Price, 2022) found that shielding had a considerable impact on mental health, with those defined as clinically extremely vulnerable having a greater likelihood of experiencing depression, anxiety and loneliness. These findings were supported by some of the participants in our research.

Twenty-two participants mentioned receiving a letter from the government advising them to shield. Some were unsure whether they had received a letter, while others assumed they had to shield because of age and/or health factors. Government guidelines were often described as 'confusing' regarding who should shield, prompting us to group our participants into four categories: first, those who shielded because they received the letter from the government in March 2020; second, those who had not received the letter but decided to shield because they felt vulnerable; third, those who shielded because a partner or child was seen as vulnerable; and, fourth, people who did not shield regardless of their particular health issues.

Douglas, for example, reported feeling 'devastated' upon receiving his letter:

'When I read the letter, and saw the text, I actually cried; I sat here on my own in my apartment. … And I'd heard about these texts going out, and I thought, they won't include me in this, I know I'm HIV positive but I've no viral load, and generally I'm healthy. When it said, you cannot leave your home for 12 weeks minimum, I actually wept; the thought of that really did affect me mentally … at the time it seemed an eternity.'

Similarly, George, a White British man who lived alone, expressed shock at receiving the letter and how it made him feel more scared of going out: "I had a letter saying that I was of the age [he was 71] that it was more, how did they put it? I was more susceptible to get the Covid virus." For George, the letter advising him that he was at risk greatly diminished his confidence about going out of the house. He was already isolated prior to the pandemic but still ventured out occasionally to the local shops using his mobility scooter, something which he stopped doing after receiving the letter. Others reported surprise about being described as 'vulnerable'. Layla, a 56-year-old Black Caribbean woman, received two letters:

'I thought, oh, God, I'm vulnerable and it was a bit of a shock because I don't see myself as being vulnerable, but obviously, the realisation that I have got underlying illnesses that I need to be aware – well, I'm aware of but that it was, I needed to protect myself from getting – or reducing the chances of getting Covid. So, that was a bit of shock.'

Some participants assumed they had to shield despite not receiving an official letter, such as Irene, an 85-year-old White British woman: "But it hasn't been a government thing with us, it's been like a communal – like everybody in the community all over the world has got to stay in at certain points. In 20 weeks, I have only been out four times. And it's awful." And Maliha, a 59-year-old Pakistani woman, commented: "I'm an asthmatic but did not get a shielding letter, my husband is a diabetic with a heart condition and he did not get a letter either but we are shielding for protection."

These comments demonstrate how our participants interpreted government advice differently, depending on their personal circumstances. They also show how, in some cases, shielding made them reflect upon their own vulnerability. The findings also suggest that the pandemic may have a long-term impact on the way certain groups of older people think about their health and well-being, long after the restrictions associated with social distancing have been removed.

Figure 4.2: Woman cooking

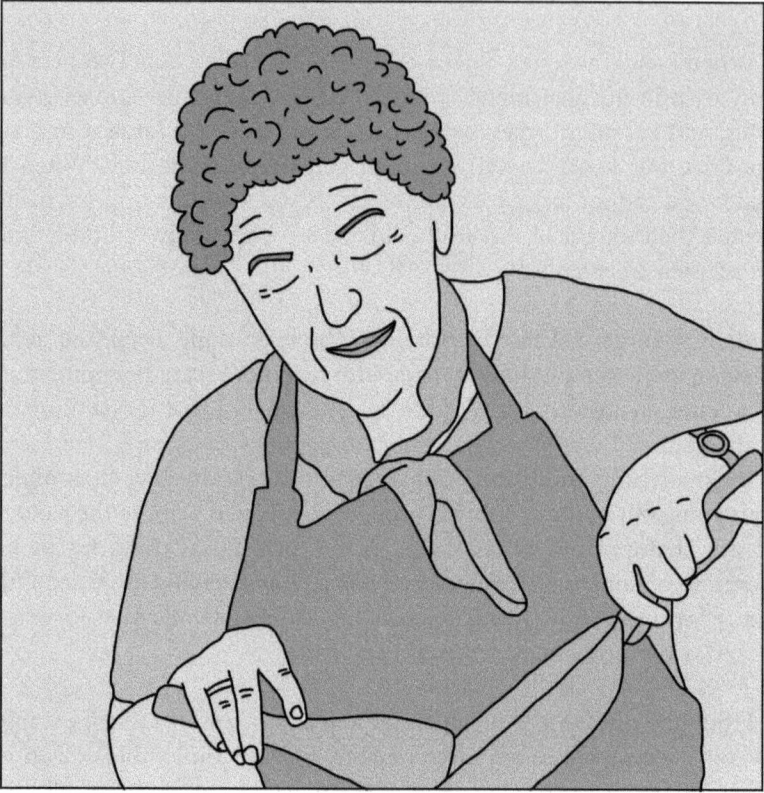

Maintaining routines

Despite the perceived difficulties associated with managing their lives, many of our respondents, highlighted the way they had tried to maintain their usual routines, in some cases developing new interests and hobbies. Saamita, a 60-year-old Bangladeshi woman, living with her daughter and grandchildren, commented: "Every day I sit at home and do my own thing, doing my prayers, housework, cleaning, cooking." Religious practice was also important for Idris, a 56-year-old Bangladeshi woman, who said she had "mainly been at home ... focusing more on my spiritual well-being. During the lockdown I spent time with my grandchildren, watched Heritage TV and connect[ed] via Zoom during Ramadan with the family."

For others, managing the lockdown was about doing more of the things which they had done in the past. Betsy, an 82-year-old living alone, had some "tapestry that's been, it's sort of getting that way where it's getting a bit boring to do but I really must finish it". Doris, an 86-year-old, found a new preoccupation: "I've got a bit obsessive now, I go around the house, scouring the house, I wash this, I wash that, that could do with a wash. So basically, where I might have washed twice a week, I have been washing every day." Miranda, an 84-year-old Black Caribbean woman who suffered from arthritis, high blood pressure and diabetes, remarked: "I am here [in the house] most of the day. I just read or do my crosswords and stuff like that. I have got a cat that gives me enough trouble anyway."

New activities and spending more time enjoying existing hobbies was also important for some of those interviewed. Phil, a 69-year-old White British man who lived with his wife had "picked up plans that I was working on to learn to play the piano so at least part of the time I am following an online course to learn how to play the piano". Some respondents described how they now had the opportunity to spend time on creative endeavours such as writing poetry, singing, doing line dancing on Zoom and making crafts of different kinds. These activities provided important ways of occupying time and (in many cases) coping with living alone (see also Fancourt et al, 2022).

Figure 4.3: Woman with laptop

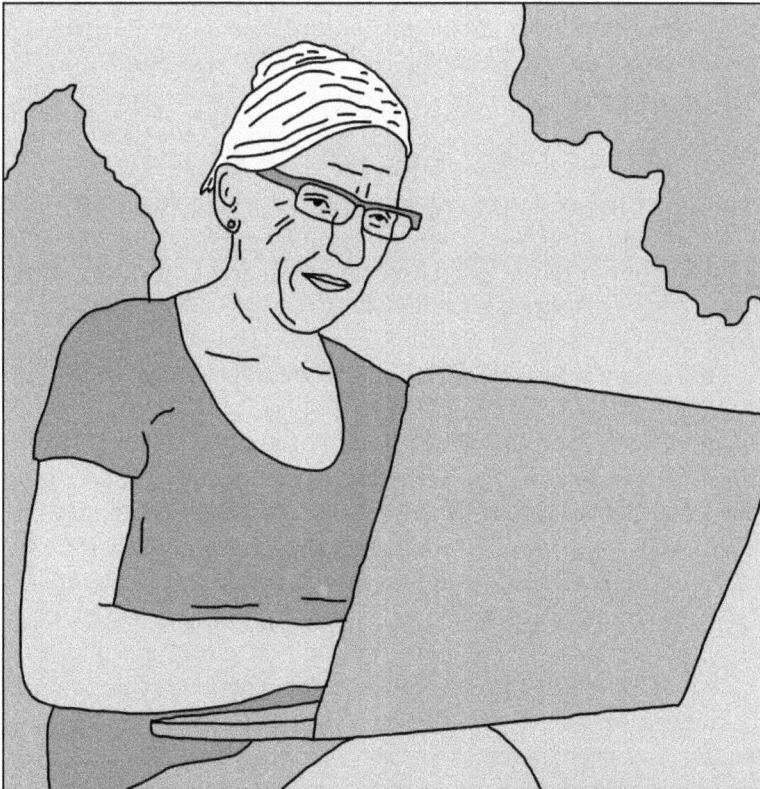

Patricia, a 75-year-old White British woman living alone, was part of a group called neonatal knitters who made clothes for premature babies. At the time of the second interview, she reported that they had "piles of stuff stacking up" because hospitals were not allowed to take the clothes because of COVID-19. Still, they carried on knitting, viewing it as both a way of passing time but also helping others. Other participants provided similar examples. Betsy, an 82-year-old White British woman, commented that: "I can understand why some people get depressed. And they do say that there are a lot of people getting suicidal, but I must admit I am not that way inclined because I find something to do, at the moment I have been knitting mini-snowmen for Christmas." Also, Pallavi, a 61-year-old Indian woman, described how:

'For a while, when I was really down ... the things I always enjoyed like knitting, gardening ... I stopped everything. So my cousin got me involved in this new online class with a group of women. I am learning new stitches. It is interesting. I have tried tie and dye too and it is promoting recycling so you have to use stuff in your home.'

In contrast, in the first interviews carried out in the spring and early summer of 2020, other interviewees commented that they were much less active compared to before the pandemic. Irene, an 85-year-old White British woman, commented:

'I'm reading but I don't sleep, and I think it's because I'm bone idle really, to what I used to do, I'm doing nothing. I'm doing nothing at all. ... They're only little things, but they're not, they're not big things really. It sounds rubbish when I'm telling you, but I'm telling you the truth. Can you imagine what it's like after being able to go out, on a coach or go shopping, or go to another town and shop, go on a train? ... I'm living but I'm only living, I'm not enjoying it.'

And Douglas, a 65-year-old White British man, commented: '[T]he thing is I don't feel productive. You know it is like sometimes I think, "Oh the day has gone and what have I done today? I have done nothing." It is like Groundhog Day, you know Groundhog [Day] when every day is the same?' Monica, a 76-year-old Black British woman, captured the sense of monotony experienced by some, as follows:

'I phone people that I phone, and then I just do a bit of gardening. I do knitting, I watch television. I go for a walk sometimes. Yeah, that's about it. You've got to repeat yourself over and over. ... The lockdown, you're locked down for six months ... you're just sitting down, you get up, you have a cup of tea, you sit down again. You've done the same routine. And you look through the window, and you sit down again … I feel locked in, and I just feel locked in and you know. … You don't know what's at the end of the tunnel.'

Shopping under lockdown

Getting access to basic necessities such as groceries became a significant challenge for many during the lockdowns. Some were dependent upon home deliveries; for others, there were concerns about entering shops with the possibility of exposure to the virus. Especially during the early phase of the pandemic, shopping was reported as arousing considerable unease, with people using words such as 'apprehension', 'anxious', feeling 'uncomfortable' and 'cautious'. There was also anxiety about the behaviour of other shoppers: people lacking regard for 'other people's health'; not 'respecting social distancing'; or 'not wearing masks'. As a result, the ordinary experience of shopping was transformed in the context of the pandemic. People had to 'rush around' rather than take their time; 'had to plan ahead and restrict the number of items [they] could get'. They also missed the 'simple things' like going into the supermarket café; or were 'put off by the queues and the restrictions'.

Views such as these were voiced across the 12-month period of research, but were particularly noticeable during the first lockdown. Eric, a 60-year-old White British man with a number of health problems (he had had a heart attack three years prior to the interview), commented: "It's very frightening at the moment … we're still a bit apprehensive going shopping. … We try and get in and get stuff and get out as soon as we can. We don't feel comfortable shopping. … We only go out to shops if we have to." Dorothy, a 78-year-old White British woman living alone, concurred:

'I think it's made me very cautious, of not, like on Thursday we decided, we'll go to Sainsbury's, and my friend is a bit, she's older than me, a few years older than me, and I said, we'll go to Sainsbury's, when I was turning out to go I was very, very anxious.'

Rushnik, a 74-year-old Indian man who suffered from depression, remarked: "You get a bit anxious you know, like you go to the supermarket and you think, oh I'm going into this bay, and then there is another five people there."

These were some of the experiences and reflections reported by our participants from two repeat interviews carried out in 2020. We return to examine this period later in the chapter when we look at more general comments about the impact of the pandemic, and explore other issues in Chapters 5

Figure 4.4: Shopping at door

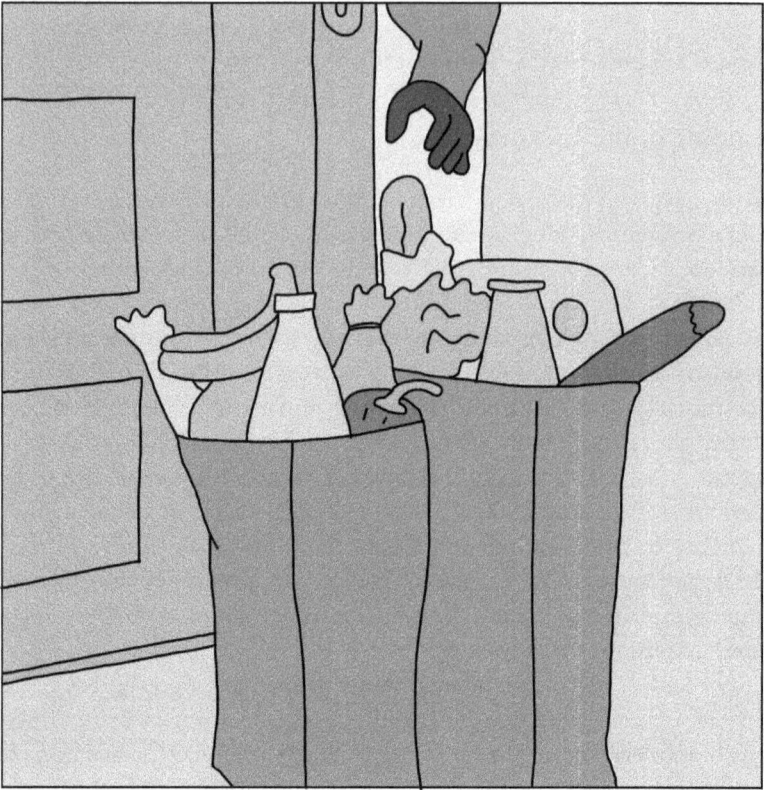

and 6. But it was clear that very few of our interviewees were untouched by the social consequences of the pandemic – whether in terms of their separation from friends and families, the disruption to everyday routines, or the impact on their own mental and physical health. The next section picks up the lives of our interviewees from the beginning of the third lockdown in early 2021, examining both their reactions to, and their more general experiences of, living with COVID-19.

Christmas under lockdown

'Given the early evidence we have on this new variant of the virus, and the potential risk it poses, it is with a heavy heart that I must tell you we cannot continue with Christmas as planned. ... The Christmas rules allowing up to three households to meet will now be limited to Christmas Day only, rather than the five days as previously set out. ... I know how much emotion people invest in this time of year, and how important it is for grandparents to see their grandchildren, and for families to be together. So I know how disappointing this will be, but we have said throughout this pandemic that we must and we will be guided by the science. When the science changes, we must change our response.' (Prime Minister Boris Johnson, Address to the Nation, 19 December 2020)

The uncertainties around the Christmas period in 2020 elicited various responses from our participants. In the case of England (outside London), three households could meet and form a 'Christmas bubble' on the day itself, restricted to a private home, a place of worship or public outdoor spaces. Our participants reported varying experiences of coming together or having to stay away from family, friends and neighbours on Christmas Day. Nikita, a 62-year-old Indian woman who lived alone and had children who she would normally have seen at Christmas, nonetheless "had a better Christmas and New Year than I anticipated as my friend who is my bubble invited me for a Christmas meal, otherwise I would have been on my own". Reema, a 56-year-old Pakistani woman who lived with her husband and two children explained: "We spent Christmas at my niece's together – it was such a nice change. We never thought before just how you would appreciate these times! It used to be normal to meet others but now it is really special."

Dorothy, a 78-year-old White British woman whose husband was living in a residential care home, reported that her "friend came to say with me from Christmas Eve. We had ... well obviously quiet like everybody else. But we had lovely food. And we were nice and warm. Next door came in just to wish us happy Christmas. And then yes it was very nice". And Betsy,

Figure 4.5: Having a cup of tea

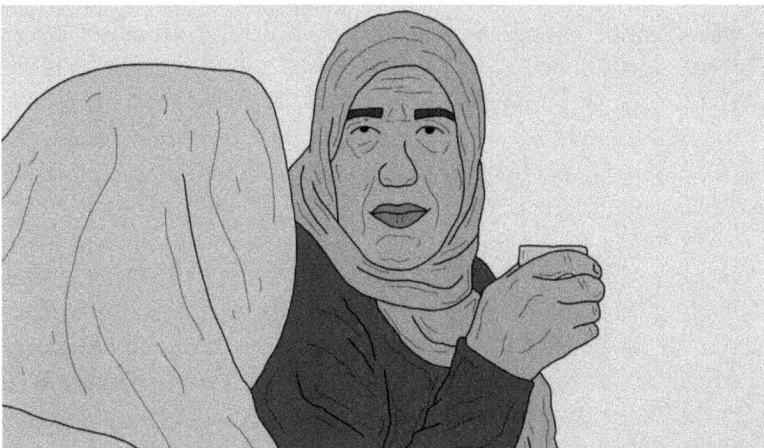

a White British woman aged 82, went to one of her daughters' on Christmas Day: "They came for me. I spent Christmas Day there. Normally I would go Christmas Eve and stay overnight but I didn't stay over this Christmas because they didn't recommend it … so I just went for Christmas dinner and came home in the evening."

But for some of those interviewed, Christmas had been a difficult period of separation from family and friends, one which brought out deeper feelings of isolation. Bhumi, a 68-year-old East African Asian woman, felt that: "It [had] been challenging to spending holidays on our own without our son and his family and extended family. It was a very lonely and sad experience being stuck at home." Daksha, a 62-year-old Indian woman, commented: "It's usually a happy time with family and friends. But this year, it did not feel like Christmas and New Year. No family came round." And Carl, a 65-year-old White British man who identified as gay, lived alone and was estranged from his family, spoke for many when he commented: "Christmas itself is such a big day where you feel everybody is having fun; and you're feeling lonely. So, I felt that particular day I needed somebody, and I was lucky in that I was able to arrange that, but I found the loneliness the most difficult thing."

As well as the positives and negatives, there was simply the novelty of a pandemic Christmas, with new and often strange routines and behaviours. Doris, an 86-year-old White woman, lived with her son who has a learning disability and has three daughters who lived close by. She recalled the Christmas period as "very awkward … nobody could come. … My oldest daughter did my shopping … she rang the bell and then went onto the drive and said, 'That's your shopping'. … It was really odd". Maxine, a 63-year-old White woman, saw her mum who lived in a residential care home for the first time since March but wearing "full PPE [personal protective equipment]". And there was the reinvention of Christmas via social media. Nadine (81-year-old White British woman) has children who lived abroad, but on "Christmas Day we did a Zoom breakfast"; Eric (60 year-old White British man who identified as gay) participated in a Christmas service: "We did it on Zoom"; and Sidney (73-year-old White British man living on his own) managed to arrange a "Zoom meeting with his sisters" on Christmas Day.

The announcement of a third lockdown, starting from 6 January 2021, did not come as a surprise to many people, given restrictions placed on households gathering over Christmas.

'As I speak to you tonight, our hospitals are under more pressure from COVID than at any time since the start of the pandemic. In England alone, the number of COVID patients in hospital has increased by nearly a third in the last week, to almost 27,000. That number is 40 per cent higher than the first peak in April. On 29th December more than 80,000 people tested positive for COVID across the UK – a new record. The number of deaths is up by 20 per cent over the last week and will sadly rise further. ... This means the government is once again instructing you to stay at home.' (Prime Minister Boris Johnson, Address to the Nation, 4 January 2021)

Soon after the third lockdown began, some eight months after the first interviews across GM, we returned to our participants to explore how the pandemic was affecting their lives. As people entered the third lockdown during the early part of 2021, two different types of experiences were voiced by many of those who we interviewed: *feeling older* as a result of the pandemic; and *physical and mental deterioration*.

Feeling older under lockdown

In the spring of 2021, coming up for a year, in and out of lockdown, some participants reported becoming more aware of their own ageing as well as the impact of time lost as a result of the pandemic. Kath, a 65-year-old White British woman, commented: "I think now people are much more thinking about death and about ... how things are finite yes. ... It is just that we become more aware of it, it may be increased awareness." Daksha, a 62-year-old Indian woman, felt that she had "[g]ot much older, have less energy, spend more time in bed and have nothing to do. Feel really lazy now, activeness is destroyed and am demotivated". And George, a 71-year-old White British man living alone, reported that: "You see so many adverts on TV about life insurance and that ... and I think, how long have I got to go, or how long has my mum got to go [to live], and it upsets me at times."

In some cases, awareness about ageing was prompted by a sense of physical and mental deterioration. The three interviews with Irene, an 85-year-old White British woman living alone, trace the changes affecting her everyday life, from August 2020 to January 2021. In the first interview, she described how she often had lunch in the communal garden of her sheltered housing scheme with neighbours who were part of her support bubble. Interviewed towards the end of October 2020, with restrictions on household mixing affecting GM still in place, Irene reported that one of her friends in her bubble had caught COVID-19 and she felt "cheesed off" because they could no longer see each other:

'So ... because I'm on complete shutdown I'm having no visitors, the only people I'm speaking to is by phone. ... No one is allowed in unless it's a medical thing and you have a carer coming, no it's complete isolation. ... At the present time I'm not eating very much, I'm losing my appetite as well, it's not the same is it when you're not seeing anyone?'

By the third interview, at the end of January 2021, Irene reported that she was suffering from long COVID and that her health had deteriorated:

'It was hard work getting into the shower because I'm just tired. The worst thing is my voice is not as strong, I can't do as much. But I'm an old lady now, anyway, so I couldn't do as much with my age, I'm 85. But I've always been a young 85.'

The cumulative effects of social distancing were summarised by Ruth, a 90-year-old White British woman, in the following way:

'All I want to do is go outside and go for walks or walk around the shops. I mean when you go for walks, you meet people who say hello to you, which I like, just say good morning, things like that. Pass the time of day with them. So, you don't feel as alone then. Because the thing I have found about not going out and not talking to people sometimes, you forget how to talk to people.'

Physical and mental deterioration

Increasing physical deterioration was a particular concern among those with mobility problems. Denise, an 88-year-old White British woman who lived alone, reported that she had lost confidence about walking because of the lack of opportunities to exercise: "I want my independence back, if I can get it and I know that a lot of it is up to me, I've got to start moving and exercising even if it's only a little bit, no matter how much it hurts." And Monica, a 76-year-old Black Caribbean woman, commented:

'I used to go to the park, yes. But I find it difficult now to walk. I don't know what's going on. I'm finding that since the lockdown, I'm really struggling. I go for walks, but I can't go as far as I used to go because I've got to walk back, and I find it difficult sometimes, walking back [home]. My legs seem to be not working as they were before.'

Participants also spoke about experiencing mental deterioration, often as a result of being confined to the home and pressures associated with providing care (see Chapter 6). Vaneeza is a 63-year-old Pakistani woman who lives with her husband, daughter and son. Over the course of the three interviews, she conveyed her increasing sense of desperation: "I'm doing housing chores, cooking, cleaning, talking to my children on the telephone and keeping myself busy in prayers. ...We didn't visit our family and relatives on our Eid ul-Fitr this year which has never happened in our lives." By the second interview, she reported a sense of "[f]ear because of this social distance we can't shake hands or hug each other, and we are always going to have this fear inside. We are so scared of human beings and I never imagined in my life that anything like this was going to happen". And interviewed for a final time in early 2021, she said:

'Most difficult is for me is that all the time staying at home is affecting my mental health which is getting worse day by day. Sometimes I put things somewhere and I forget where I put it. I really want to go back to my country and meet my father, relatives, and my cousins. Then I will be in peace.'

Reflections on the impact of lockdowns and social distancing

How did our participants reflect on how their lives had changed over the period of the research, given the changes which had affected their daily lives? Much of the discussion and research on experiences of the 2020–2021 lockdowns has focused on their negative impact, especially for those with limited resources, and/or subject to different forms of discrimination. But among our own participants, there were contrasting views and reflections on their everyday lives during the periods of lockdown. For some, they had provided space to reflect upon their lives, to appreciate their time with family, or to establish a new sense of priorities. Nabajit, a 70-year-old Bangladeshi man, commented:

'I've always been outgoing and very extroverted, but this coronavirus gave me a sense of purpose. Made me think, who am I? What am I doing? And what I'm going to do. So, I question myself, I get plenty of time to address my own fears. That has given me a new kind of discipline. I have enjoyed my life now, the last leg of my life, and now I'm very tranquil and also in peace with myself.'

Kath, a 65-year-old White British woman, also commented on the benefits of spending more time alone:

'Though I was ill, the first few weeks of lockdown was amazingly peaceful. Yes, I loved, you know, the fact that you couldn't hear the traffic, you could hear the birds singing. It was really beautiful and also [I was] much more centred inside myself. ... I did notice that during the time of the proper lockdown that it was easier to notice things, to feel ... life a lot more easily.'

For others, the lockdowns reaffirmed the importance of family relationships. Sharon, a 53-year-old Black British woman, felt that:

'More bonding, together with my husband and my children. So, we are more happy to be together all the time. Yeah. Bond with all my children, because before this lockdown, we don't think about doing Zoom. We be waiting for, oh, are we travelling down [to see her daughter]? Because my fourth daughter, she lives in Dublin. We looking for, oh, we travel down before we see each other. But now, two ways, all the family we do Zoom. ... Then I have more time for my home.'

Bhakti, a 51-year-old Sri Lankan woman, echoed Kath's view:

'It's [the lockdown] made me realise that how much I actually enjoy my own company, because I've kept sane ... and it's made me realise who my real friends and who my real neighbours are ... there have been a lot of positives that have come out of it. And I think for people generally, and I just hope that some of the positives, the way people treat each other and we look out for each other, I hope that continues ... like everybody you have your down days; but those days thankfully have been few and far between, I think there have been more positives than negatives to this experience, thankfully.'

But the other side to the impact of the pandemic must also be acknowledged, namely, the sense of 'fear' and 'panic' which it aroused among many of those interviewed, a theme which came across most clearly from some of the respondents drawn from ethnic minority communities, groups who had been among the worst affected from illness and death from COVID-19 (see Chapter 2). Cameron, a 56-year-old African-Caribbean man, worked as a nurse and had direct experience of the impact of the devastation wrought by the pandemic: "[T]o see people dying every day, the numbers going up, it's not coming down. ... The most difficult like I said before is the panic."

Azhar, an 83-year-old Pakistani woman, commented: "I felt scared, feared for my daughters and their children. I also have become paranoid and kept telling my grandchildren who lived with me not to come near me." This experience was also mentioned by Pallavi, a 61-year-old East African Asian woman living alone, who reported: "I felt like I lost control and was isolated." Yasmin, a 64-year-old Pakistani woman, emphasised a number of these themes:

'I was so depressed. Before it was like we can visit family friends and relatives and now we are just stuck where we are. I miss a lot my mother who is sick and I can't go to visit her because she is in Pakistan so that hurt me more than anything. Now I really don't want to visit anybody or can't meet anyone outside because of fear.'

Many of the interviews confirmed the way in which the lockdowns resulted in losing out on the pleasure and support associated with contact with friends. Patricia, a 75-year-old White British woman who lived alone, had lost her closest friend to COVID-19, and commented: "I do miss her obviously. Miss going up [to visit her] and chatting to her or whatever." Jackie, a 68-year-old White British woman, had lived with her mother for some time but now lived alone, and was frustrated at "[n]ot being able to go out and see my friends and having a coffee and having a laugh and just generally mooching around and seeing people with happy faces".

Not being able to 'hug' close friends and family was highlighted by many participants. In the first interviews, 17 people mentioned missing hugging loved ones, increasing to 46 in the third interview. Idris, a 56-year-old Bangladeshi woman who experienced feelings of depression and isolation, felt that: "The most frustrating part has been the human contact – not being able to hug my extended family or friends." Stewart, a 72 year-old White British man who lived alone and suffered from depression, commented: "[T]he single thing I most miss, I think it's just being, to be able to just interact with my friends [and] … I miss hugging my grandkids." And Patty, a 64-year-old White British woman living on her own, also singled out "[n]ot being able to hug people. Because I have no contact with my biological family and really there's no next of kin as such you miss giving someone a hug because of the social distancing, because everyone needs a hug now and again".

For some of those interviewed, there was the pressure of avoiding passing the virus on to a vulnerable member of their household. Benazir was a 71-year-old Pakistani woman who cared for her sick husband as well as her sons. She commented:

'This lockdown left me feeling on my own. All services were limited. This made me angry and upset. I had so many questions. I was used to a walk every day to maintain my mental health, get fresh air and stay sane but that had to be avoided as I was scared, I don't want to pick the virus up and end up giving it to my husband or sons.'

Paula, a 75-year-old White British woman living alone who identified as gay, also described the dramatic effect of the pandemic on her life:

'I felt scared, I felt really scared … it has changed me because I don't feel I'm as light-hearted as I feel – I'm a heavier person in terms of – I've never had this – I've never been a person that has been depressed, ever. I've never felt depressed, but the lockdown, I have felt more down than I have ever felt in the whole of my life.'

The impact of bereavement

A major source of stress for our participants, increasing in its impact over the course of the research, was the loss of family and friends as a result of the pandemic. The psychological costs associated with the toll of bereavements has yet to be fully acknowledged, with at the time of writing (September 2022) over 200,000 deaths in the UK due to COVID-19 or involving the virus. As Rosen (2022) notes, 200,000 is '[a] lot of deaths for us all to cope with'. In the period covered by our research, people experienced the loss of the rituals associated with funerals, and regretted not being able to provide the support and practical assistance they may normally have given to bereaved friends and relations. Such everyday formalities and informalities associated with loss and mourning are woven into the fabric of daily life. Over time, their absence, or the extent to which they were heavily restricted, may have substantial consequences for individual health and well-being as well as for relationships within families.

In our research, the death of family and friends was a feature across all of the phases of the interviews. However, experiences of bereavement were more common over time and were a particular feature of the interviews carried out in the early part of 2021. Frank, a 76-year-old White British man living alone, described how:

'2020 is my annus horribilis, the terrible year. I lost three important people in my life ... John was at the beginning. John was a very good friend ... a very good neighbour ... I used to call him my soulmate. ... It is a great loss. I miss him greatly and I still get a bit upset when ... I'm getting a bit upset now talking about him.'

Cameron, 56-year-old African Caribbean man, who is married with three children, felt that:

'The most difficult thing is friends that you know that are dying, which you know, last week there two of my friends they all passed, they all died. ... For the past one month between now and the beginning of the year, I will say about four or five people [have died]. It was very bad to me, when I think. So, it made me feel a bit down because someone that you know, a close friend that had died and I couldn't even be at the funeral.'

Zahra, an 81-year-old Pakistani woman living alone, was supported by her son and daughter-in-law. She explained:

'My daughter-in-law has been telling me some my friends have died due to COVID … it really scares me. The more I hear about the increase in death rate the more fear is built up inside. I struggle to keep positive. I am losing friends to COVID daily and this brings upon my anxiety.'

Jackie, a 68-year-old White British woman living on her own, explained how upsetting she found watching news about the pandemic:

'In the beginning I had quite a few bad days when I felt quite sad and weepy, I could see all these deaths coming up and these people, family don't have the opportunity to say goodbye and the things about the funerals and that, only eight people, if you know what I mean, you can't hug anybody. I thought that was quite sad.'

And Pallavi, a 61-year-old East Asian woman living alone, talks about the impact on Christmas celebrations:

'My mum passed away just before Christmas so there was all sorts of mixed emotions really. It was the first time without my mum but I was also excited to see my dad and the little ones but sad because mum wasn't there. Very strange and emotional. I couldn't go to her funeral so it was the first time I had seen my family in a while.'

Pallavi's excerpt illustrates the complexity of the social dimensions of the pandemic: joy at seeing her family after a period of separation but an event suffused with the incomplete mourning of the death of her mother; a day of celebration becoming linked with the process of grieving. Little wonder that people just wanted to return to living 'normal lives': a view expressed across each of the three interviews carried out in the study. Irene, an 85-year-old White British woman, spoke for many when she said:

'It will be a relief just to know that if I want to go and visit my friend, I can do instead of waiting for a phone call or making arrangements. If I want to go out shopping and one of my friend's calls or my family calls, I can go with them. If we want to go out for a meal, say, let's go out for a meal tonight – if we only go for a chip and fish café meal, we've gone out. I think it will be a great relief, just to be able to be normal.'

Anwar, a 51-year-old Pakistani man, agreed: "I think everybody's waiting … just coming back to the normal as soon as possible." And Ruth, a White British 90-year-old woman who lives alone, also commented:

Figure 4.6: At the seaside

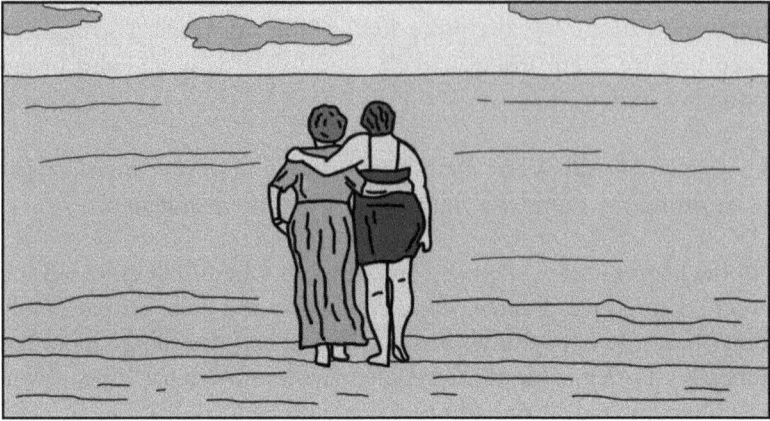

'I mean when you're on your own and you get to a certain age you do feel, you feel lonely. Because all your friends, your sisters and brothers, everybody is gone, all my family … you're still going to feel lonely because the thing with people who you knew when you were younger, they know you, they know what you were like. People who see you now only see an old person.'

She described her hopes for the future, commenting: "I think everybody's thinking about things like … walking at the seaside. … It's just like a dream. I've just got it into me head I want to walk. … Paddle in the sea, I don't care whether it's cold or not. Once I get there, I'm going to do it."

Conclusion

This chapter has described a period of a year in which the lives of most of our respondents were changed beyond all recognition. Simple routines such as shopping became more fraught as people worried about 'catching the virus' in crowded supermarkets. Restrictions were placed on socialising, which exerted a toll on relationships, whether or not being able to 'hug' friends and family, meet for coffee, or enjoy a family Christmas. Some of those interviewed felt changed as a person – 'feeling older' as a result of the lockdowns; having 'much less energy'; or feeling less physically or mentally able or 'deconditioned' as it came to be termed (Public Health England, 2021).

Yet it is also the case that people 'made do' in various ways: keeping up existing hobbies or finding new interests; in some cases spending more time on prayer and reflection; or just doing a lot more housework and – especially in the first lockdown – spending a greater amount of time in the garden or other outdoor spaces (see Chapter 6; also Fancourt et al, 2022). Running through all these experiences was also the constant reminder of the toll of illness and death from COVID-19, with the daily mortality rate provided by the media something which many of our respondents found especially difficult to bear.

From this overview of the different experiences found among our respondents, across the three waves of interviewing, we now illustrate the issues raised in more depth, by exploring four case studies and relating people's responses to the virus in the context of their individual biographies and key turning points over the course of their lives.

5

Experiences of the pandemic: a biographical and longitudinal analysis of four case studies

Introduction

Chapter 4 explored experiences across all of the groups of participants, revealing a variety of responses to the lockdowns over the period 2020 through to early 2021. Analysing these themes further, this chapter discusses how experiences of the pandemic were shaped by the nature of people's lives prior to the onset of COVD-19. Many of the interviewees mentioned key biographical *turning points* which influenced how they experienced or viewed the impact of COVID-19. For some, it was a mental health crisis, the separation from, or death of, a spouse, or an incident resulting in long-term unemployment. For some of our gay participants, turning points related to reactions to 'coming out' from their family and friends. As well as, in some cases, deepening a sense of precarity in later life, these turning points also provided some of the participants with resources to cope with the challenges brought about by COVID-19.

A case-study approach has been chosen in order to provide a detailed analysis of the 'holistic and meaningful characteristics of real-life events' affecting the lives of our respondents (Yin, 1989: 14). This approach enabled us to explore a complex set of experiences in detail and to recount the role of life events *over time* (Feagin et al, 1991). The interviews were analysed longitudinally, examining how responses changed (or stayed the same) from one interview to the next, per case. Four individuals were selected purposively from the groups in our sample, in order to examine different dimensions of everyday life. They include: *Carl*, a 65-year-old White man, who lived alone and identified as gay; *Frank*, a 76-year-old man, who lived alone in a flat in a high-rise building; *Raquela*, a 50-year-old Black Caribbean woman who lived with her aunt during the first lockdown; and *Soraya*, a 54-year-old Nepali woman who lived with her extended family in north Manchester.

The following analysis takes these four cases in turn, and explores how life-course circumstances influenced people's reactions to, and experiences of, rules such as those associated with social distancing. The participants entered the pandemic through contrasting pathways, drawing on a range of resources and strategies to cope with what proved for many a transformative period of their lives. The discussion draws together themes across the cases, and examines different aspects of time which appeared in the interviews, including: key moments in the life-story, changes to everyday life over the three interviews, and perceptions of ageing. To conclude, the discussion shows that some participants were able to draw on previous life events to help them cope during the pandemic, while others had greater difficulties, due to their already precarious lives.

Carl

Carl is a 65-year-old retired manager of a charity, who lived alone and identified as gay. He was in a long-term relationship for 30 years, but his partner died nine years previously. Discussing his life history, Carl described a crucial turning point in his early 20s, when he came out as gay, and was subsequently rejected by his family: "I have a brother and sister who have not spoken to me in 40 years ... so, basically, I have no family members, I only have a family of friends that I've made and so I've become quite a resilient person." Despite facing considerable adversity, Carl emphasised that he had a fulfilling life with work and volunteering: "And so, having that full life I have to rely on my resilience really of being a strong person and trying to see the positive side of things."

Carl felt that the pandemic had affected him "mentally more than physically". In the first interview, he commented on the problem of living alone and knowing whether you are ill with COVID-19 or something else: "It's difficult when you're living alone ... sometimes and you get a bit of illness and you don't know whether its mild symptoms, you know, whether it could be the virus, you get a bit anxious and worried about it." Interviewed two months later, in July 2020, he lamented not being able to see a close friend for some time, saying: "And I really miss, well, miss him but just miss the fact that I can't do ordinary things when I want to do them and that is what makes me feel a bit down." Carl had been hoping to "bubble up" with this friend but, six months into the pandemic, this had not happened: "So, I've been very lonely and isolated over the last period." Six months later in January 2021, Carl described how his relationships with friends seemed to have become more distant: "Just because you're not seeing people face-to-face. Simple things but they haven't felt so simple, like just meeting a friend and having coffee, and having a catch-up, you know it's very difficult."

Prior to the pandemic, Carl was heavily involved in various social activities, including volunteering at an HIV charity, an advice centre and a group which supported older people who identified as LGBTQ+. Since the lockdown, Carl had been trying to keep the group together through emails, text messages and phone calls, particularly for people living on their

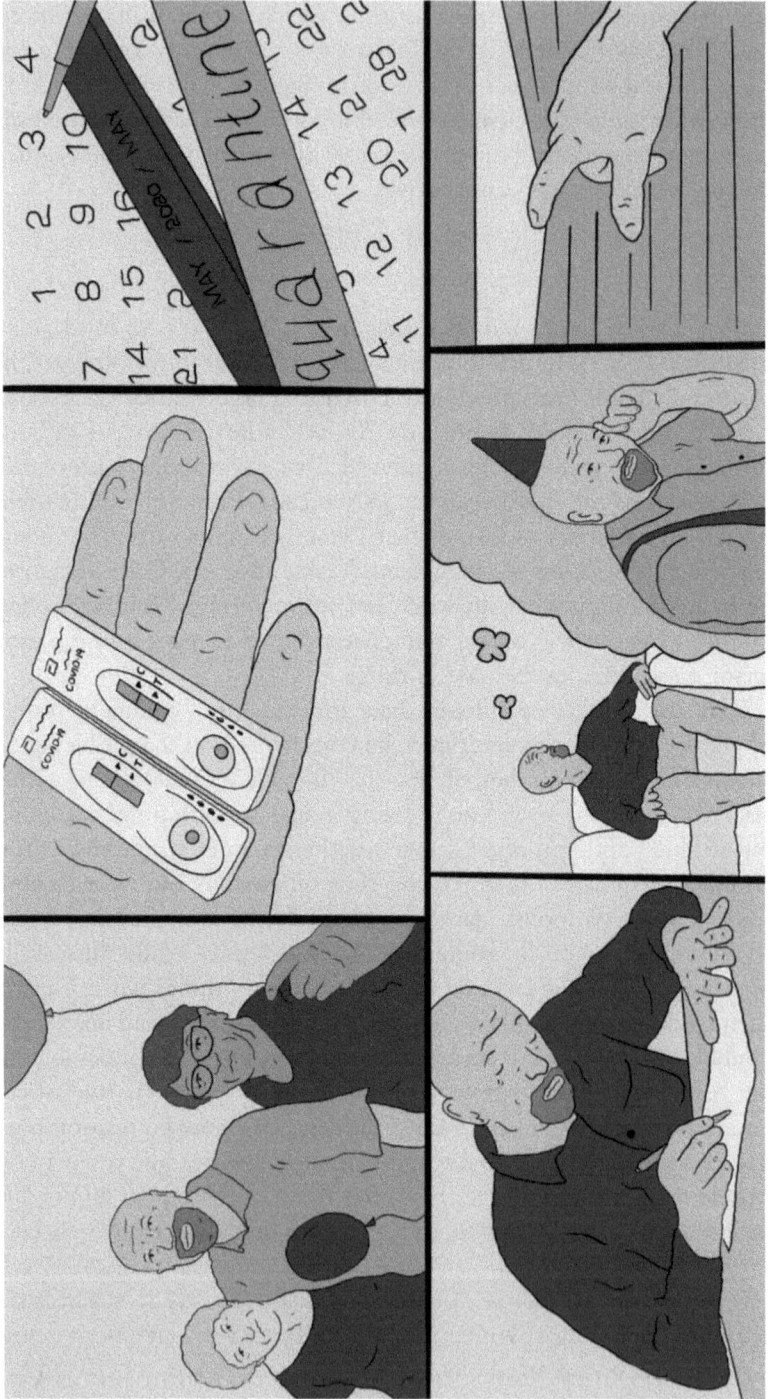

Figure 5.1: Carl's story

own. He mentioned that "[S]ome of us in the group have discovered new skills, for example FaceTime". Carl also used Zoom but explained how unsatisfying it was:

'When I've done things like Zoom meetings, I've found myself more depressed afterwards. I don't know what's happy about it. I know it's all we've got at the moment in many cases, but I just felt like you're not seeing the real people, and you're not – I mean I know some people really like it, but I know quite a lot of people who do find it difficult, and I'm one of the people, I just find it very difficult.'

In his second interview, Carl commented how prolonged periods of time at home made him feel "lethargic". The lack of face-to-face contact had not been compensated for by Facebook, email or other means of communication. He also missed volunteering, which was an important part of his identity and provided continuity with his previous work role. Carl commented on the significance of his friendship network in the context of rejection by his family of origin. He commented: "I've been very, very lonely, and isolated over the last period." Carl was concerned about the long-term impact of the pandemic on his relationships. He described how the loss of a friend and family member had a profound impact on him:

'I had a bit of depression for a few days when a friend of mine died. It was somebody I used to work with and we were very close. … I mean, I haven't seen him as much since I retired but he's still a friend and it affected me quite a lot when he died. And I sent some money towards the funeral costs because I wasn't able to go. And also in the same week, an auntie died who was 92. And I'd written her a letter which I knew she'd received before she died but I wasn't allowed to go to the funeral because they would only allow seven or eight people. So I felt, you know, upset for a few days. But in general, isolation, you know, I wouldn't like the rest of my life to just be like this and not thinking, oh, at some future date we're going to get back to normal, we're going to be able to meet, socialise and have fun and laughter. I'm missing all that sort of stuff, that's how I feel in my head, it's affected me much more mentally.'

Reflecting on the impact of the three lockdowns, Carl commented on the extent to which his positive attitude to life had changed. He explained:

'Before COVID, I was sort of happy-go-lucky, a relaxed person and now I feel a lot more anxiety and a lot more worried about things, but I am trying to look forward to the future with positivity that we'll get the vaccine, we'll get out of this, life will return to normal and I can get back to volunteering, back to socialising and what feels like a normal life where I am in control of what I want to do.'

Carl described how he had always been "quite a resilient person, you know someone who can get on with whatever is thrown at you and I have always been somebody who can enjoy my own company". Usually he liked living alone, but the pandemic had made him realise how "isolated" he had become, which had a dramatic impact on his health: "I've not been trying to lose weight, I've lost two stone in weight." Carl attributed his weight loss to anxiety:

'I've been seeing the GP and they're trying to sort of just monitor me to check and have blood tests and things to see if everything is OK, but it's had a big effect on me emotionally. I've been very anxious and it's not like me because normally I'm a very sociable person, I do a lot of volunteering and I've had to drop that obviously because of COVID, you know, these things have stopped happening.'

Overall, over the three interviews, the decline in social contacts, and losing friends and relatives over the course of the year, made Carl feel increasingly vulnerable. Despite having an extensive friendship network, he felt increasingly isolated leading to the new experience of feeling lonely (see also Vlachantoni et al, 2022). Prior to the pandemic, Carl felt well supported by a circle of friends connected through a social group for LGBTQ+ people. He relied heavily on his friends since being rejected by his family in his 20s and losing his long-term partner. Carl's life-story shows how events, such as coming out, which create precarity in one period of life, may help protect an individual from vulnerability later , as shown in Carl's case where he talked about his strength and resilience. However, during the pandemic, Carl started to feel more negative about life and increasingly conscious of the disadvantages of being a single man living on his own.

Frank

Frank is a 76-year-old man, who has lived alone in a flat in a high-rise building in an inner-city neighbourhood in Manchester, for 15 years. He had been retired for many years after having a varied career, including working as a librarian and a psychiatric nurse. As with Carl, a central theme to emerge in the interviews concerned mental health pressures arising from the pandemic. However, unlike Carl's busy social life, Frank explained how he was practically housebound before the pandemic, due to numerous health problems. He had received a letter in March 2020 instructing him to shield,

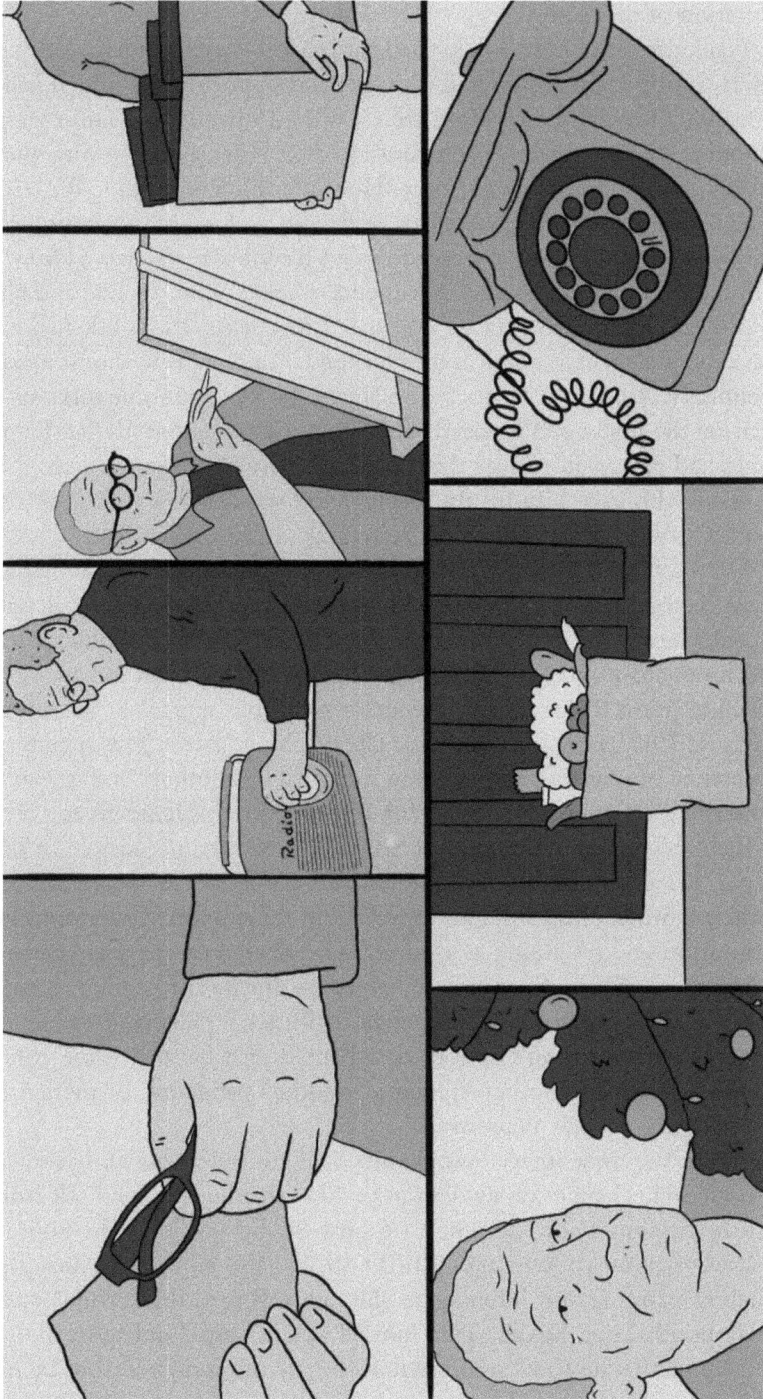

Figure 5.2: Frank's story

due to his "multi-morbidities", and he had not left the house during the duration of the study.

Frank described how he had tried hard to feel "happy with his lot" in terms of accepting his more limited activities and opportunities which had been a feature of his life even before the COVID-19 pandemic. Throughout the duration of the project, Frank continued to enjoy spending time pursuing his interests and hobbies at home. He was confident looking for resources online and had a strong network of friends and health professionals who he felt he could call upon if needed. But his interviews showed how being confined to the house had a detrimental impact on his mental and physical health, resulting in feelings of isolation. Even before the pandemic, most of his time was spent at home as he explained: "I was getting almost locked-in, voluntary." But since he started to shield, he became more anxious about leaving the house and worried about letting anyone into his flat. Frank had only had two visitors over the 12-month period of the research, a health worker who gave him his flu vaccine, and the other, a volunteer assisting with COVID-19 vaccines who he reluctantly let into his flat.

Discussing his life-story, Frank described himself as a "working-class Salford lad" and spoke with regret about leaving school with no qualifications. An accident on a building site early in his working life left him in chronic pain and with mobility problems. The accident was an important turning point in his life, a "precursor of all my mental health problems, because I had a breakdown, basically, not long after". This precipitated a sequence of negative events; "one thing led to another" and it resulted in "breaking up my marriage". Frank reflected on this incident as a moment which changed the direction of his life, for better and worse. On the one hand, it led to a mental breakdown and the loss of his marriage; on the other, it provided an impetus to reach out for support, going onto further education and retraining as a nurse. He reflected on these experiences to make sense of his worsening mental health during the pandemic and what he saw as a positive shift in societal attitudes: "[T]hese days, if you say 'depression', you don't have to be ashamed of it because – the pandemic alone has caused another epidemic, another pandemic of mental health problems, especially depression."

Across the three interviews, Frank's daily routines were fairly similar, but a noticeable change was evident in the way that he felt about self-isolating. In the first interview, he described how he did not leave the house as he felt wary about contracting COVID-19. He also enjoyed various pastimes such as painting and listening to the radio. But in the second interview, two months later, he described himself as "reclusive" and agoraphobic. He explained that he had "mood swings" before the pandemic, but he realised that something more "sinister" was going on after spending prolonged periods of time alone. In the third interview, around eight months after he was first interviewed, in February 2021, he described how over Christmas he had been very ill and his doctor prescribed antidepressants.

Frank's narrative indicated a fragile social network although he said he was close to his three adult children. One daughter visited regularly, dropping off shopping at the front door, as he was shielding. During the interviews, he apologised for talking so much, explaining how much he missed chatting. In the third interview, Frank lamented losing touch with friends over the years, and described how 2020 had been a "horrible year". He had lost three close friends, one was a "fit bloke" who had died from COVID-19. Frank described how he regretted not telephoning him more regularly. Frank also found out that his daughter had been taking money from his bank account when she was withdrawing cash to pay for his groceries. He said that they were still friends, but he was deeply upset and shocked: "I thought, if you can't trust your own daughter … who can you trust?" Frank had not discussed it with her but said that he had forgiven her as she had problems with debt but it was an unpleasant episode: "[B]asically meant that I had to sack her, it wasn't nice."

Frank missed seeing friends and family, but did not like speaking on the telephone or using Zoom as both made him feel anxious. He talked on the telephone once a week with an old friend, as well as to his family. Frank also spoke regularly to his GP and a link worker who provided support with his mental health. In the third interview, Frank explained how he found calling people difficult, describing it as "phone-aphobia". He explains that sometimes he would nearly have a panic attack:

> 'Well yes, again, I've lost a lot of people because of it. Obviously, they feel that I'm ignoring them – well, I am in a way – but I don't mean to do it. I mean, people that I was very fond of and got very friendly with, once I left I stopped phoning them and then, after a while, they stopped phoning me – that's how it happens.'

Overall, Frank was already living a precarious life before the pandemic, due to his long-term physical and mental health difficulties. Throughout the three interviews, his daily routines were fairly similar, but a noticeable change was evident in the way that he felt about self-isolating. Over the 12-month period, Frank became increasingly anxious and distrustful. He found communicating with friends and family over the phone stressful, and was worried about the added strain of the pandemic on his close family relationships.

Raquela

Raquela is a 50-year-old, Black Caribbean woman who worked as a community activist and interfaith minister. Prior to the pandemic, Raquela

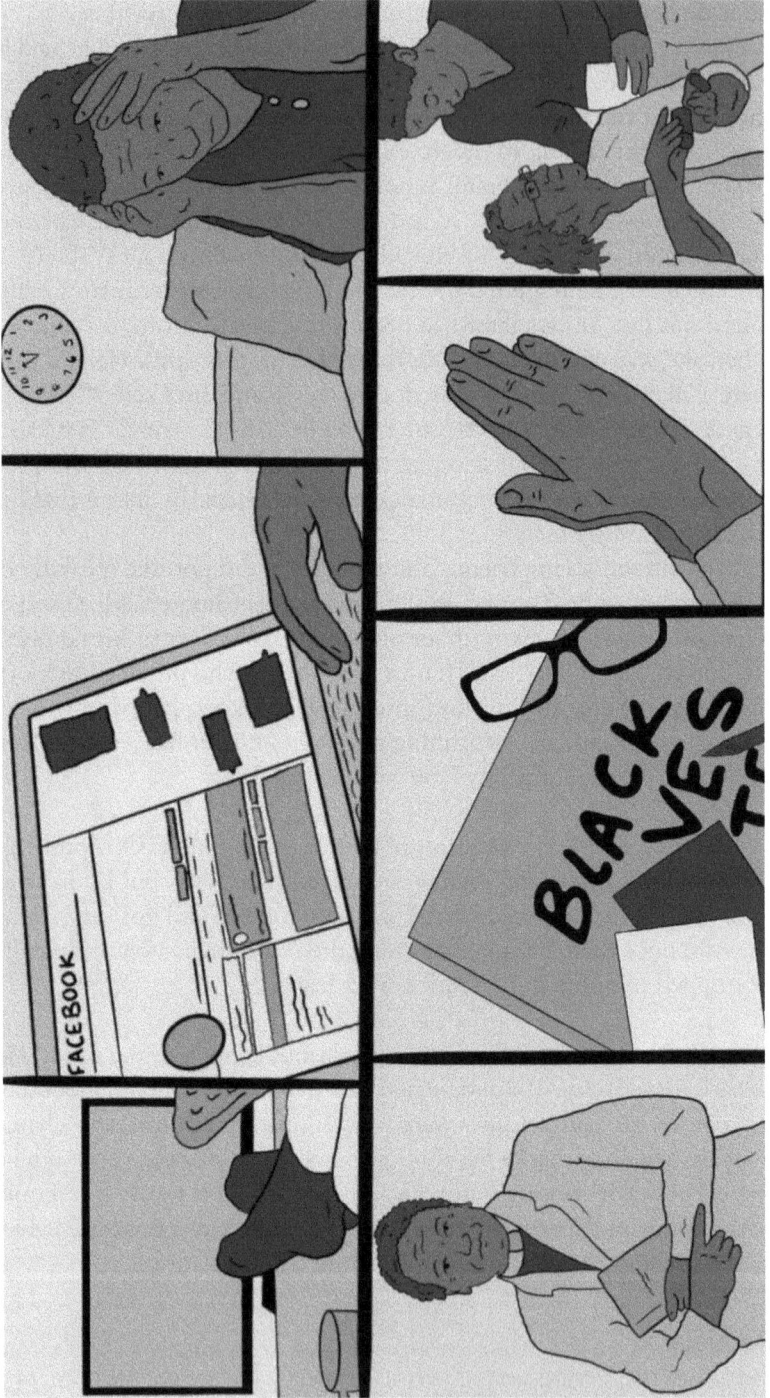

Figure 5.3: Raquela's story

lived alone in north Manchester but at the time of the first interview, she was staying with her aunt, who was unwell, to support her during lockdown. A theme which ran across the three interviews was the unequal impact of the pandemic on the Black community. Raquela stated: "The saddest thing for me was we lost so many members of Black people in the Caribbean community."

Discussing her life-story, Raquela explained how she was born in Manchester and was brought up by her Caribbean grandmother, as her parents could not take care of her. She described how she was a "high-school dropout", and went on to have two children as a single mum. Asked about what impact her upbringing had on the rest of her life, she explained:

'I think that it's made me have an outlook on life a little bit different. And I think that there's almost a part of me that, I think if I did live with my parents, I wouldn't be able to do the things I do for people and be the way I am in life. However, there has been times when I, you know, experienced depression and anxiety and I do think that when them times are here, I do think that some of that is to do with my parents.'

To help overcome the difficulties she faced in life, Raquela commented on the importance of faith: "[M]y personal relationship with God I think is very strong and I'm in constant prayer and conversation with him. He's been the same God since I was young, the God that my grandmother taught me and where I went to church." Prior to the pandemic, like Carl, Raquela had a busy social life: "I would meet friends and usually go out for lots of meals or I'd cook for them or they would cook for me. I like to go out dancing, so, maybe every couple of months we would go and hear some soul music and dance." She described how all of these activities came to an abrupt stop, and how she missed contact: "I'm a big hugger. And so, there's no hugging no more. I've been really renowned for my hugs … it's really damaging human beings because we're not used to it and that's not how we function."

Two recent turning points for Raquela were incidents involving the police, which occurred during the first lockdown and which she had reported as acts of racial harassment. These incidents had a profound impact on her mental health, resulting in periods of anxiety and depression: "I couldn't sleep, and I wasn't eating." Another important moment for Raquela was the Black Lives Matter protests, which spread around the world in June 2020:

'My life was quiet, I would sleep quite late and I just called it holidaying at home at first, in the first many months. … The first three months, I'd say. … Up until Black Lives Matter happened, it was very much – we were holidaying at home, there was lots of Netflixing, lots of clearing out a little bit, lots of lazy days. I was catching up with things that I couldn't do before. But it was a quiet time and there was the odd meeting and the odd Zoom, but nowhere as much as after Black Lives Matter.'

From this point, political activism became the focus of Raquela's life, taking up "much of my space and my time". Raquela also commented on the death toll caused by COVID-19 among the Black community: "[W]e've lost a lot of members of our community, especially since Christmas, and you're looking at five or six a week, sometimes two a day." She explained:

'You go on Facebook and it's like, "I've lost my mum, I've lost my dad, my brother". There was one picture that they showed, and it had about eight men in it, and four had gone [passed away]. ... One of them was my cousin's dad. And what I'm conscious of, so what I'm mindful of, I keep sharing gratitude, because I'm waking up every day. The pain, even in the unsettledness and I'm noticing that I'm also grateful that I've got my health and I've got my second bubble here. I just keep being mindful that I'm eating every day. There are so many people that are not waking up, that are not eating, I keep finding that I'm constantly sharing gratitude, really.'

Raquela's interviews revealed some interesting reflections about her plans for the future as she wanted to "challenge" herself and do something new. Prior to the advent of COVID-19, Raquela had decided that she would like to go overseas and volunteer. She described how she had "no strong commitments" in Manchester, as her sons had both moved out of home. However, she explained how as a result of COVID-19 her plans had been changed:

'What's happened since COVID is a group of people have come together and because of COVID they're trying to build a co-housing [scheme]. They're looking for members. So, I've been in touch with them already because do you know what ... I'm out in the sticks in Tameside and I don't know anyone there. What I've realised is I need to be near the family. ... And I feel like COVID has brought this to me like, this is the change that's going to come because life is never going to be the same again and I've always wanted to live in co-housing, and I'm 50, and to me this is the perfect time to do this. It would be almost like an investment for the rest of my living years.'

She explained how the co-housing group was formed because of the experiences of people living during the pandemic: "If COVID hadn't happened I don't think that group would have formed. And they've said that it was COVID, experiencing COVID that they then realised that they wanted to do this." In the third interview, four months later in February 2021, she had enrolled on a degree course and was making plans for the future. Raquela saw the lockdowns as a moment to reflect and think about the future anew. She commented that the pandemic provided an opportunity to take stock:

> 'I've listened to people's concerns around Covid, but spiritually for me, there was something about – we were meant to stop. ... And we were meant to rest, and we were meant to look at our lives and we were meant to rethink our choices and do things differently when we come out.'

Overall, throughout the 12-month period, Raquela dedicated her time to caring for her aunt and was heavily involved in community activism, spurred on by her own experience of racial discrimination, and the high death rates witnessed among the Black community. This case suggests that some individuals used the pandemic as a unique period for self-reflection, helping to preserve their well-being during the pandemic. Raquela was determined to make something positive from the changes brought about as a result of the pandemic and planned ahead for a new life involving travelling and moving to shared housing.

Soraya

Soraya is a 54-year-old Nepalese woman who lives with her husband, two sons and grandson in a rented house in north Manchester. Before the pandemic, she worked as a waitress. Like Frank, Soraya suffers from long-term health problems, including diabetes and depression, both of which were exacerbated during successive periods of lockdown. She kept in regular contact with her family in the UK and Nepal using social media: "I use WhatsApp mostly to get in touch with my family and friends but a few times Facebook for my few friends who are back home." Over the period of the study, she commented on how much she missed seeing her friends, and felt increasingly isolated and depressed.

Across the three interviews, Soraya's daily routines remained fairly similar. In the first interview, in July 2020, she stated: "I love to spend my time cooking, cleaning and offering my prayers. Sometimes I like to watch TV. I do spend time on social media like using Facebook and YouTube." Although she regularly used her mobile phone and social media to talk to friends and family, Soraya missed seeing people face-to-face. In particular, visiting other homes, sharing food, going shopping and taking day trips: "We can't meet people, we can't go out for hoteling and we can't go in gatherings.

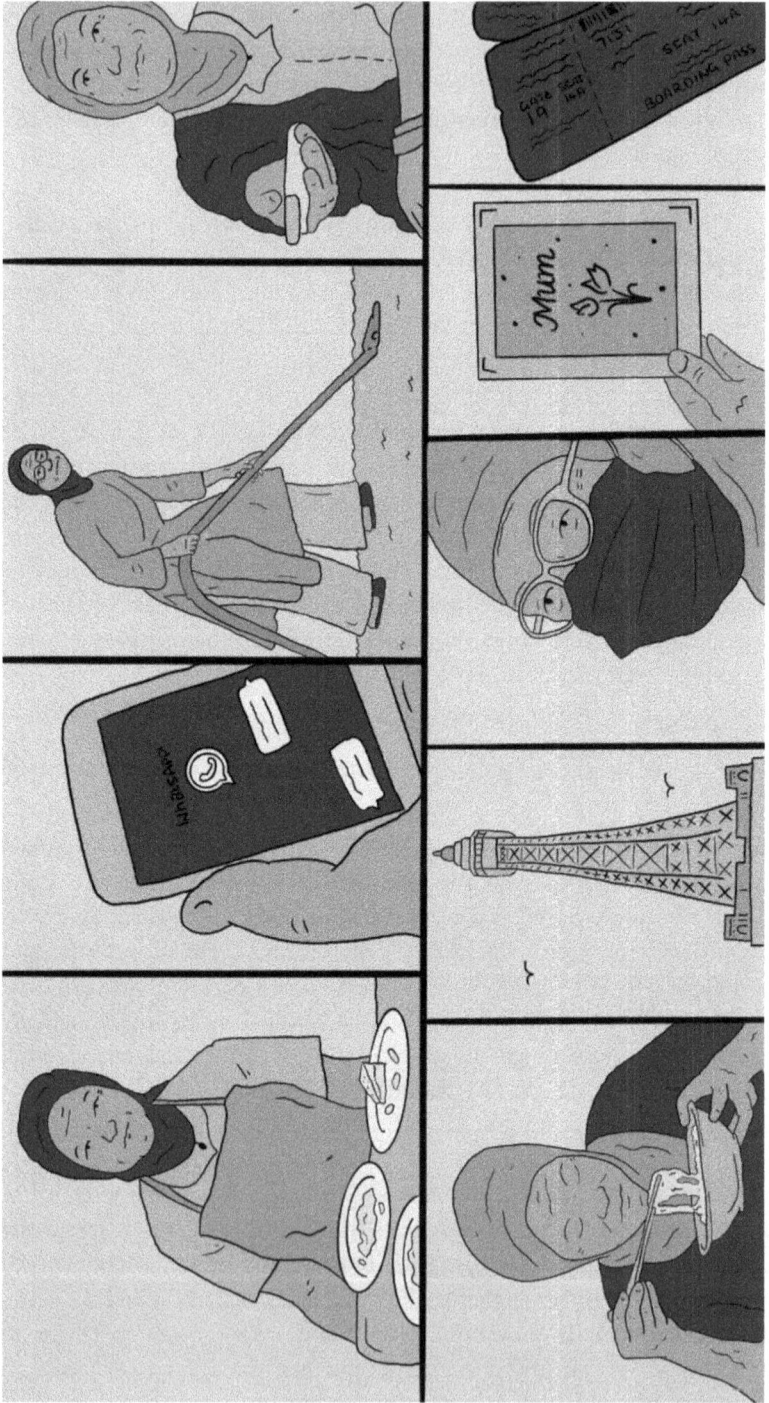

Figure 5.4: Soraya's story

We have to stay at home and it's so depressing." Being at home for extended periods made her feel anxious: "All the time staying at home is so boring and depressing. Before lockdown when we used to go out, it makes us [feel] fresh but in lockdown staying at home all the time makes us so tensed."

At the time of the second interview, in November 2020, lockdown restrictions had been eased and Soraya enjoyed spending more time away from home. Reflecting on the loosening of restrictions, she appeared to be more optimistic: "Things got better and many places got opened like markets and restaurants. Now human beings got a bit of freedom so they can go around freely." Asked about her coping strategies, she explained that her daily life was monotonous: "Mostly I spend my time on cleaning and cooking. I like to spend my time in praying and reciting Quran. So everything is same like before and nothing has changed." Despite stressing how her routines had largely stayed the same, she added that she was "working less" in the house and enjoying socialising more with friends. She had also been away on a weekend trip to Blackpool with her son.

Yet despite seemingly having more freedom, Soraya explained how the restrictions continued to have a negative impact on her mental health: "The rules of lockdown make me fed up and I got tired of following those. I have so much fear when I'm about to meet people and going into a social gathering even if it's our families." Like Carl, Soraya longed to socialise again, as she had done before the pandemic: "I hope to have same like before because we used to exchange foods and going each other house which I miss a lot now." Discussing the possible end to restrictions, she said: "I hope this happens and it is such a good news. We are going to have less tension, stress and feel more free. I think that our lives are going to be very easy."

In the third interview, carried out in February 2021, Soraya described how the lockdown during the winter had been particularly challenging. She hated the cold and staying at home "all the time". She missed her old life and described how the stress had impacted upon her physical health:

'Nowadays I am developing a new habit which is forgetting things as I am diabetic, [also high] cholesterol and blood pressure. Everything [cholesterol and blood pressure] is high, and there is no way to make it low even though I'm not eating much. Main reason is staying home then because of that I start thinking too much which leads me to sadness.'

Like Frank, Soraya was caught in a negative cycle of isolation, mental stress and physical ill-health. Looking ahead, she said that she did not have many plans, but was greatly looking forward to being able to "finish with this lockdown and we come out from this depression of which is the cause of staying home all the time". Soraya was very anxious about contracting

COVID-19 due to her underlying medical problems, describing how she had "so much fear" about the disease. When she left the house she always wore a face mask and washed her hands on return. But she found wearing a mask uncomfortable: "I find it so difficult wearing mask with glasses because whenever I put mask on then my glasses got steamed so I have taken it off and clean then put it again. I also started having breathing issues with wearing mask."

Soraya explained how she felt scared to go out during the first lockdown, but in the second interview, felt a bit better, "but I still I have this fear of Coronavirus. Because in my family three people died from COVID-19 and my brother, sister and my niece, they have been to hospital caused by COVID-19". A particularly difficult event for Soraya was the death of her mother:

> 'She was ill and she was inviting me to meet but I couldn't go just because of this lockdown. I was very close to my mother and I couldn't meet her in her last days, this regret is going to be with me forever. ... When there wasn't any lockdown and my mother used to be ill. I used to go straight after hearing about her illness but now just because of lockdown I couldn't see my mother's face in her last time.'

Reflecting on the future, Soraya was concerned about the long-lasting impacts of social distancing. In particular, she was worried about a deterioration in relationships: "This coronavirus is always going to stay in our minds even though we will go through [other things]. We are going to go far away from each other and I really don't think that we can be normal again as before." Soraya also talked about how many lives had been lost during the pandemic. In the second interview, she explained: "We are going to die before our time comes. We are not going to live our lives with freedom and life is going to be very hard." The phrasing, which is translated, is interesting. The pandemic made Soraya think about the finite nature of life and whether or not living with restrictions is truly any sort of life at all. Soraya longed to travel again and visit her family: "Travelling is on my top of list. Yes, it has changed a lot because it has been so long that I didn't meet my siblings and close family members who are back home." Her isolation was particularly pronounced. Soraya reflected on the interview by saying that she was pleased to have had the opportunity to talk to someone about her experiences: "I feel good to share about lockdown because usually we don't talk about it."

In Soraya's interviews, she made a number of comments which indicated how her relationship to her home was rather complex. For example, in the first interview, she described how the night before, the neighbours were very noisy which had meant that she could not sleep. As a result, "I spend my all day spent in tension and depression. Now I feel like I should take antidepressant and go for sleep. I couldn't do any house chores at all." In the second interview, she explained how even though she lived with her extended family, she often felt lonely, describing: "Everyone is so busy and no one have time to sit with anyone. My one son comes home and another goes to work so we hardly get time to sit on table for food. Sometimes weeks that we didn't even see each other." Therefore, these findings show how Soraya's sense of home was rather complex and ambiguous. Her home was a sanctuary from the virus, but at the same time, she felt frustrated and lonely spending prolonged periods of time there.

Overall, Soraya's life did not change much during the 12 months, and her faith remained a central coping mechanism. While she lived with her extended family, she felt lonely, and even though she kept in regular contact with friends and family online she missed face-to-face contact, particularly visiting friends' homes and sharing food. Soraya became increasingly isolated and anxious over the 12-month period and was concerned about the long-lasting impact of the pandemic on her relationships. Her feelings of isolation also had an impact on her physical and mental health, as she struggled to manage her diabetes and depression.

COVID-19 and the life-course

The four cases illustrate how experiences of the pandemic differed greatly between individuals, depending on their life-course circumstances and daily life prior to the pandemic. The longitudinal analysis reveals the following cross-cutting themes across the four individuals.

First, exploring the life-stories of the participants demonstrates how events and behaviours at earlier life-stages have consequences for later life, in particular on relationships and well-being (Bengtson et al, 2012). As a result, COVID-19 can be placed in the context of biographical turning points, such as being disowned by the family (Carl), mental health crises (Frank) and bringing up two children alone (Raquela). The findings support Settersten et al's argument that older people place events such as the pandemic in the context of 'a broader range of experiences ... [to] judge [their] relative significance' (2020:4). For example, Carl, who was rejected by his family in his 20s, fostered a degree of resilience from past experiences to cope with the challenge of being forced to isolate during the pandemic. Likewise, Frank made sense of his worsening mental health during the pandemic by reflecting on problems experienced earlier in his life, especially relating to an accident he had on a building site.

Second, the longitudinal data draws attention to continuities and changes which the participants experienced over the 12-month period of the study. Across the three interviews, Frank and Soraya's daily routines were fairly similar, but changes regarding how they felt about self-isolating were evident, with feelings of disconnection from social ties increasing over the successive periods of lockdown. Their experiences reveal how already-lonely adults often inhabit the intersection of different types of vulnerability, in our examples long-term health problems, mobility issues and restricted activity (Bundy et al, 2021). For example, Frank's physical and mental health problems worsened as he was unable to leave the house. Similarly, Soraya felt that her medical problems had become difficult to manage because she was exercising less for fear of contracting the virus, creating a downward spiral in her mental health.

Carl and Raquela were quickly able to move their volunteering activities online, which provided them with a greater sense of continuity to their pre-pandemic lives. For Raquela, her political activism provided her with a sense of purpose and solidarity with others. In contrast, even though Carl continued to communicate with members of the LGBTQ+ community through Facebook and Zoom, he felt that these interactions did not make up for seeing people in person and contributed to his feelings of depression. Supporting Fuller and Huseth-Zosel (2022) findings, during the pandemic, some older people felt that technology did not contribute to good quality social connections. Despite using online platforms to communicate regularly, Carl and Soraya both commented on how they were deeply concerned about the long-term impact of the pandemic on their relationships.

Existing research shows that those who live alone, such as Carl and Frank, are at the greatest risk of isolation (Portacolone et al, 2021; Willis et al, 2022). Single men and widowers are especially vulnerable, as older men may not be as embedded in family and social networks and long-standing relationships (see Chapter 6). Our research supports these studies, and demonstrates how both men reflected on living alone in a new light, due to the pandemic. Carl did not have a family network to support him but strong friendship networks played a crucial role in providing 'not only ... emotional support but also ... practical and economic support at times of crisis' (Heaphy and Yip, 2003: 7). The analysis of Soraya's interviews also shows how people living within extended family households may also experience isolation. Even though Soraya had a strong family and friendship network, she felt lonely, and increasingly tense, confined to the home. She also worried about the long-lasting impact of the pandemic on relationships.

Third, all four cases show how older people who were forced to 'shelter in place' during the pandemic felt a loss of independence (Settersten et al, 2020: 5). The participants felt frustrated by the lockdown rules and longed to be able to return to their normal pastimes and routines. Raquela was anxious to embark on a new chapter in her life. She described how she had gained some "freedom" at 50, as her children no longer needed her, but how her life was on hold due to the pandemic. Over the 12-month period, Frank and Carl reported becoming more aware of the passing of time, and their own ageing. In Soraya's and Carl's cases, awareness about ageing was reinforced by a sense of physical and mental deterioration arising from the impact of successive lockdowns (see Chapter 4).

Conclusion

This chapter explored four case studies from our qualitative longitudinal interviews, revealing insights into the impact of the pandemic over 12 months. The analysis supports Portacolone et al's (2021) argument that COVID-19 may amplify insecurities which people had in their lives prior to the pandemic, especially those relating to health and finance. For the participants discussed here, the pandemic exposed the fragility of pre-pandemic lives, and the challenges faced in dealing with the crisis associated with COVID-19. In some cases the pandemic introduced *new vulnerabilities*, exacerbating the already precarious lives of some of those interviewed. For example: Frank became further isolated as he was fearful about using the telephone as a means of communication; Carl described how he was in good health before lockdown and felt well supported by a network of friends, but that prolonged periods of time on his own had affected his mental and physical health. The participants were also concerned about how their relationships would suffer in the long term and whether the pastimes and daily activities they enjoyed before the pandemic would ever resume.

6

Changes in relationships

Introduction

COVID-19 and the subsequent lockdowns led, for most of our respondents, to significant changes in relationships with family, friends and neighbours. Rules on social distancing produced, as already explored in Chapters 4 and 5, significant adjustments to everyday life, from the inclusion of temporary lanes inside supermarkets, to avoiding close contact in public spaces. At the same time, intimacy also emerged in unexpected ways, as in the case of befriending services that multiplied during the pandemic, or in different types of support provided by friends and neighbours. This chapter explores how social and caring relationships were reorientated, what impact this had on older people, and the factors behind these changes. The discussion is organised around five themes: *increased social isolation*; *pressure at home*; *changes in contact with neighbours and in the neighbourhood*; *outdoor spaces*; and *the role of technology*.

This chapter uses the idea of 'landscapes of care' to consider the different spaces through which caring relationships were experienced and maintained, as well as the spatial patterns that emerged due to social distancing. Through an analysis of how the social relationships of our participants changed during the course of the various lockdowns, this chapter will show the importance of space and place to these relationships, and the new spatial arrangements of care that emerged during the pandemic.

The concept of landscapes of care is used to provide insights into where care occurs and the complex spatialities that care relationships entail (Milligan and Wiles, 2010). In the context of this study, this means thinking about the ways in which people renegotiated their relationships *within* different spaces of care. Such landscapes may involve the institutional, the domestic, the familiar, the community, the public, the voluntary and the private, 'as well as transitions within and between' (Milligan and Wiles, 2010: 738). Landscapes of care also encompass 'networks of care' – the social relationships between individuals and groups – and the infrastructure that support such networks. The concept is used to aid understanding of how relationships and networks changed during the pandemic, as social distancing altered people's engagement with their social networks. The discussion begins by exploring the impact of the pandemic on a group who were found to have relatively fragile networks of care – single men living alone.

Increased isolation: the case of single men

One of the most challenging aspects of the COVID-19 pandemic concerned the restrictions on social interaction, notably during the three periods of lockdown covered by our research. The longitudinal approach adopted revealed both how some groups of people felt more isolated over time, and how the urge to connect made people explore new horizons and technologies. Social distancing produced feelings of isolation across many of those interviewed in the study. However, for some of our participants, reduced contact with friends and family was part of a pattern set before the pandemic, one which seemed especially characteristic of the 21 men (out of the 49 interviewed) who lived alone.

George was a 71-year-old White British former factory worker. He had been out of work for over 30 years as a result of a bad back and lived alone in a housing association flat. By his own account he was already isolated prior to COVID-19, but lockdown had meant that he stopped going out altogether. In his first interview, he commented how he had started "shutting [himself] away", a response reinforced through the closure of the communal garden in the housing scheme. In his second interview, George remarked on what he saw as his physical deterioration, commenting: "Sitting down a lot has really crippled my back in a way. My back was bad but it has got worse with not exercising ... they haven't opened the communal room for some time." Interviewed for a third time, three months later, George expressed additional concerns: "It gets very lonely at times even though I have carers come in. ... I have put on a lot of weight, I'm 21 stone now. And I have trouble standing. It's hard to make it out to the kitchen, just to make a cup of tea."

Figure 6.1: Making tea

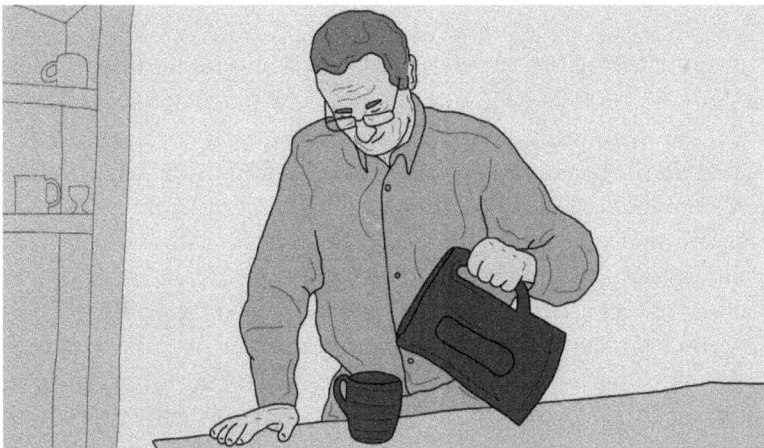

While George had a close relationship with his step-daughter and step-grandchild, he said that he had no friends and carers treated him "as though I'm an idiot". In George's case, his sense of isolation increased due to health problems and a limited social network. He voiced concern about the impact of having even less mobility in the future and how, because of his tinnitus, he felt unable to join activities conducted over the telephone or online.

Another example of the type of isolation affecting some of our participants was illustrated by Simon, a 58-year-old White British man who had never married or had children. He was born with a physical disability, and used a mobility scooter to get around his neighbourhood. His first and only job was as a labourer but he had been on disability benefit for a number of years because he was unable to stand for long periods. Simon lived on a busy road with no shops close by. As a result, he used his scooter to get to his nearest supermarket. When asked about his social network, he said he doesn't "bother with anybody". He said he had hardly seen anyone since the start of the pandemic, except when he went to the shops. During his first interview, in July 2020, Simon felt that "nothing had changed" and that he actually preferred lockdown, although he did admit missing attending his dominoes and lunch club and not being able to volunteer one day a week at a local charity shop. However, interviewed three months later, Simon reported feeling increasingly isolated, which was having an impact on his physical and mental health:

'I'm not coping very well and I'm fed up with staying in. Lockdown makes me want to drink more ... I drink 10 to 12 cans a day ... I go to the communal garden for a bit of fresh air and meet neighbours. My next door neighbours cooked me a Christmas dinner and brought it round to me front door which was lovely ... [But I] don't think I have a future ... I can't see one.'

For Tom, a 64-year-old White British man living on his own in a tower block, the pandemic had made him realise how much of his life had "shut down". Tom was greatly affected by the social impact of the pandemic. He struggled with depression and found making friends difficult: "I am not a great conversationalist to be honest ... I do not really do small talk and I have only just realised that puts me at a distinct social disadvantage." In the second interview he commented: "I had not realised how much of my life I had shut down in that sort of way really ... over the year. I have just lost my friends basically and I have not made the effort to make new friends. I need to now make the effort really." Nine months later, Tom spoke again about his desire to try something new: "I am seriously going to be looking to doing some voluntary work. I have just realised how empty my life is really … but it is something I can do something about. That is positive. … With everything shut it has made me realise how insular I am."

Sidney, a 73-year-old White British man, had been living on his own for over 20 years following the death of his wife. During that time he had developed various routines and activities to rebuild his life. However, with the lockdown he felt that everything was once again "on hold". Before lockdown, he described how: "I could go, if I had got nothing else to do, I could go and sit in one of the libraries but the library's been closed. I will sometimes … sit in a café somewhere." By the third interview, Sidney talked about how much he missed going on holiday and "wandering round places" like shops in the city centre where he would browse and have a meal, seeking out company.

In comparison, Brian, a 74-year-old gay man who lived alone in the centre of Manchester, did not see much change in his relationships except being unable to see people face-to-face: "I've been in touch with people through Zoom and Facetime, and I haven't lost touch with anybody … I would not have done this before the pandemic." Brian had good support from neighbours; he was in a bubble with one of them who helped him with shopping when he was shielding. He also felt, as a gay person, that he has a different experience of close relationships:

'People who've had their personal relationships disrupted I understand. But I don't have those kinds of relationships if you see what I mean … I think that because I'm gay, because of when I came out years ago, because those experiences of alienation and so on, over many years, I think I'm in quite a different situation compared to other people.'

In contrast, Douglas, a 70-year-old single man who was also gay, highlighted the extent to which the pandemic had made him realise the potential isolation of being single:

'Some of my friends, gay friends and straight friends, they're either married or they've got a partner living with them, and so they've got somebody else to chat to, to lean on, to talk to, share things with; and I think that must make a huge difference. And that's one thing I have felt, the kind of isolation of being a single man, 70 years old, who suddenly is cut off from all the normal social activities that he would do. So I'd say that that's had quite a big influence on me really.'

Among some of those we interviewed, single men living alone presented experiences of intense isolation. The context was one of people going into the pandemic with fragile social networks, poor physical health and low incomes. Many had found ways of 'coping' through their involvement in places such as community centres, local cafés, libraries and pubs. The additional pressure created by COVID-19 concerned the closure of these vital forms of support, the loss of which had a considerable impact, and was a reminder of the importance of their eventual restoration, especially within inner-city neighbourhoods (Yarker, 2022a).

Isolation and care in the home

Those who were living alone were particularly susceptible to feeling isolated during the pandemic. However, our research also found that living with others did not always protect our participants from feeling isolated. Changes in family dynamics, both within the home and with extended family, were experienced across our sample. Some participants reported feeling that they had become closer to their family, either because they were spending more time together at home (see also Chapter 4), or because they were in more regular contact with family members who checked on their well-being more often and offered practical support. Lakmini, for example, a 63-year-old Sri Lankan woman who worked as a cleaner before the pandemic, struggled financially because she no longer had any income from her paid work, but really appreciated the extra time with her family:

'We didn't have time to stay home before, the three of us. But now these days, we are sitting together, we have breakfast, lunch, dinner at the same time all together. We shared and we are sharing our problems to each other. It is getting better these days, because we are having a very free life, but it is also hard.'

However, for others, the pandemic resulted in more difficult changes in their relationships, with increasing pressures involved in providing care in the home. This was especially the case for some of the South Asian participants, who had previously relied upon family members and those living within the household. Fariq, a 68-year-old East African Asian man, provided insight into some of the complicated reorientations of family relationships during the pandemic. Fariq told us he had become "dependent" on his son who would deliver shopping and other essential items by leaving them outside his front door: "Even before I got COVID, I became dependent on my son to supply us with all the essential food and other personal items which were left outside the house at the front door."

These feelings of dependency increased after Fariq caught COVID-19, the result of which he felt had changed his relationship with his wife:

'I have become much less able to conduct tasks around the house to support my wife. She is my main carer and I feel frustrated not being able to assist myself and moreover, my wife. I am still in recovery, and I am not the same person any more with the long-term impact left from this virus.'

Fariq's case draws attention to the changes affecting relationships among family members and the landscapes of care within the home. Fariq had increasingly become dependent on his wife, as his ability to help around the home had diminished. In addition, both he and his wife had become cared *for*, albeit at a distance, by their son, provoking complicated feelings of dependency. Azhar, an 83-year-old Pakistani woman, also felt a sense of dependency on her family, a feeling that was increased by her lack of English and anxieties around catching the virus. Azhar relied heavily on her family for access to help, due to her not speaking, reading or writing English. Although she lived with her son and daughter-in-law, with the onset of the pandemic she became increasingly anxious about becoming ill and being unable to see other members of her family. By the third interview, Azhar started to consider returning to live in Pakistan as she found the pandemic "very mentally draining". Her anxieties were compounded by the fear of not being able to be buried in her home country if she died during the pandemic: "My most [biggest] anxiety is that flights [are] not going to Pakistan and you are not able to take [a] corpse to your home land. My wish is to be buried in Pakistan. I panicked so much that I said to my family to take me to Pakistan." For Azhar, even though she had a close network of family support at home, the possibility that she would not be buried in her birthplace was a major concern, demonstrating the close relationship for Azhar of landscapes of care both within her home and in Pakistan.

Zahra, an 85-year-old Pakistani widow who lived alone, told us how the pandemic changed her life as she could no longer go out regularly and see friends. Because she is diabetic and has high blood pressure, her doctor advised her not to leave the house. Her son lives in the same street and, during the first and second interviews, she visited her son regularly and prayed five times a day:

'Coronavirus has changed my everyday life, I used to go out and see my friends which I am unable to do. ... It's same routine day in, day out. Get up, have breakfast, watch TV, go to my son's house. I read [the] holy book every day to keep myself occupied, read my prayers five times a day.'

In the second interview, she was more hopeful and was starting to go out shopping again:

'I feel things are bit better because of some relaxing rules I can go see my friends whilst observing social distancing. ... If the weather is good I take a trip to town and spend time sitting on [a] bench, if any of my friends see me they also come and join me and we have a chat.'

But by the third interview further concerns were expressed: "My daughter-in-law has been telling me some of my friends have died due to COVID-19. It really scares me. I don't know how to use social media. ... I struggle to keep positive. I am losing friends to COVID-19 daily and this brings upon anxiety."

For some of our participants, the most profound change in their family relationships was having more restricted contact with extended networks of care. This was something that was of particular concern for some of the South Asian women in our sample, and in some cases, was compounded by an increase in their caring responsibilities within the home. For Maliha, a 59-year-old woman from Pakistan, the death of her brother was experienced not only as a personal loss, but also resulted in additional caring responsibility for her mother: "[I]t has been miserable", she told us, "painful and I have not had time to grieve. [It has been] physically, emotionally and spiritually draining".

Having reduced access to formal support networks also resulted in increasing pressures for participants such as Benazir, a 70-year-old Pakistani woman, who describes the impact that social distancing has had on her life in the following way:

'I look after my husband and my sons. I have carers who come and help me care for my husband's needs daily. I don't have a social life or any hobbies as all my time is focused on looking after them. I was struggling financially to begin with before the pandemic started, and payments were all scheduled via payment plans for all my expenses. My husband being bed-bound means more spending on hygiene products being bought and extra care to be provided. This lockdown left me feeling on my own. All services were limited. This made me angry and upset.'

By the second interview, some participants who had been involved in caring responsibilities during the lockdown reported feeling tired and an increased sense of isolation. Buhmi, a 68-year-old East African woman of Indian origin, was the main carer for her husband, and was shielding to reduce his risk of catching the virus. When interviewed six weeks after her first interview, she described her situation as having grown worse, with her son and his family now being unable to visit to provide support: "My life has become more restrictive with the recent lockdown measures in Greater Manchester. My son and his family who support us and were in our bubble group cannot visit anymore at our home or in the garden."

The excerpts from the interviews with Maliha, Benazir and Buhmi illustrate how feelings of isolation arose despite living with others and sharing busy and often overcrowded households. Such pressures were exacerbated by the increased pressures these women felt as carers. Increasing caring responsibilities at home, along with having to remain physically distant from extended family networks, led to an increased sense of precarity as a result of being cut off from important familial relationships.

The experiences of our participants demonstrate how having to remain physically distanced from friends and family was a source of anxiety and isolation for many participants, whether living alone or with extended family. Although their circumstances were very different, physical proximity with family (such as living in the same household) did not always protect participants from experiencing increased social isolation within their homes. Indeed, in some of the examples from our research, this proximity (notably for women) seemed to result in additional pressures.

Relationships with neighbours and local community

Changes in older people's relationships during the pandemic assumed various forms, with social interaction being reworked in novel ways. Intimate relations had to be negotiated to accommodate social distancing, and relations such as those with neighbours gained a new dimension. For some, the pandemic brought the neighbourhood into people's landscapes of care for the first time, and in doing so created new meaning for people in the places in which they lived. This was also a landscape that allowed older people to actively participate in caregiving themselves. However, there were contrasts in the way older people in this study accessed care in their neighbourhoods, with inclusion for some but the experience of social exclusion for others.

Boundaries between closeness and distance among neighbours are commonly marked through a process of trial and error, reflecting variations dictated by culture, class and age (Lewis, 2020). However, understanding of these boundaries was also affected by the more defined parameters set by the British government during lockdown, as well as by a collective perception that at a time of need, some people were more vulnerable than others. Where relationships of support did exist, these involved both informal networks of care between immediate neighbours, as well as more formalised networks of care involving community and voluntary organisations (see Chapter 7).

Carl, a 65-year-old White British man who lived alone, spoke of the generous support offered by neighbours from the outset of the pandemic: "As soon as the lockdown happened, one of my neighbours put a note through my door with a telephone number and said if I need any help or any shopping, to ring her number." Douglas, a 70-year-old White British man who also lived on his own, commented:

'If you're looking at the whole of the COVID period I think [neighbours] definitely got closer. People are looking out for each other and more people would knock on my door during the first lockdown and say ... "Is there anything you need from the shop?" ... They would come and help in the garden.'

The spaces outside of, and in between, individual homes became increasingly important during the pandemic. Spaces such as doorsteps, windows, garden fences and driveways became imbued with new meanings as they enabled some degree of contact with people outside the household. Such interactions often turned into more regular forms of contact and friendship. Dorothy, a 78-year-old White British woman who lived alone, said her neighbour rang her every morning: "We'll have a chat about whatever's going on, we have a laugh, and we laugh our way through it really, because it's been you know, we'd see something and we'd, we'd laugh about things, it's kept us up, or we've moaned [laughs] you know what I mean."

These neighbourhood networks translated into ways in which participants could provide care for others, as well as care for themselves. Barry, for example, was a 73-year-old White British man who lived alone and during the pandemic he had started volunteering for a local voluntary organisation delivering food: "People have helped me so, I'm trying to give a little bit back, if I can do that for half an hour for somebody, then that's great. It's only an hour a week, it's one of the times I go out." He reflected on how even spending a small amount of time helping others had really helped him too: "It makes you feel OK actually. And meeting people sort of thing. I don't talk to them, I've no time but I just say hello to them." This comment recognises that 'interdependences and reciprocity are characteristic of care relationships' (Bowlby, 2012: 2102), and in the context of the pandemic, caring for others was often perceived as being mutually beneficial. Ruth, a 90-year-old White British woman, made sure she opened her curtains first thing in the morning "so the people across the road won't worry that I'm not well" and Bhakthi, a 51-year-old Sri Lankan woman, started to exchange eggs for vegetables with her neighbours who she had only briefly talked to before the pandemic.

The need to check on an elderly neighbour who has no family nearby, or to do the shopping for another neighbour who was shielding, made some people more willing to approach neighbours. For Ray, a 59-year-old Black British man living on his own, the shift in his relationship with neighbours had been a surprising one:

'With the neighbours I didn't realise how, you know, how they look out for each other, in a sense, so that was new for me. So I wouldn't say it's become closer, it's just the fact that we were always I think,

Figure 6.2: Exchanging vegetables

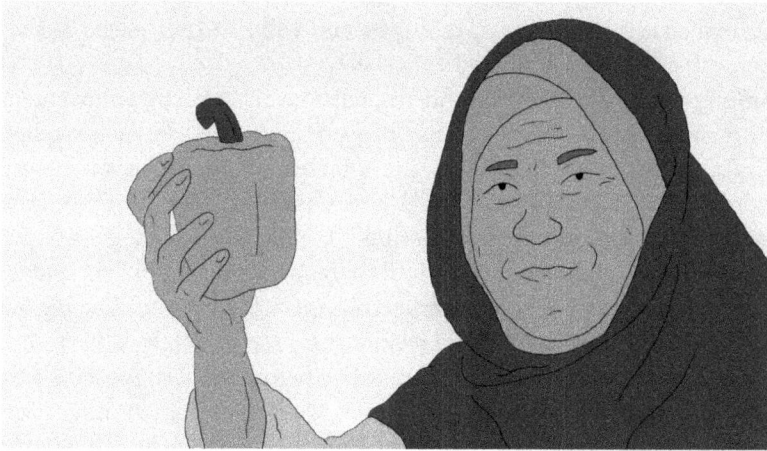

neighbourly, but the fact that they knocked on my door tells me something completely different.'

Over the course of the three interviews, we heard from participants about how they had become more acquainted with their neighbours, and how for some, clapping for the NHS on a Thursday evening during the first wave of the pandemic had brought a sense of community to their street. But the experience of neighbourhood life varied considerably among those who we interviewed. In some cases, interviewees reported hardly ever seeing neighbours, as in the case of Jackie, a 68-year-old White British woman who lived on her own: "I don't see my neighbours at all, I've seen a new one that's moved in, but they tend to be very transient around here, they only stay about six months and then they move on to different areas ... the community is being lost over a long time."

While sources of community support were much celebrated during the pandemic, it is important to remember that this was not the experience of those living in transient or what were experienced as hostile neighbourhoods (see also Lewis and Buffel, 2020). Some respondents described feeling alienated from their neighbourhoods. For example, Raquela, a 50-year-old African Caribbean woman who was spending time away from her home, looked after her aunt in a neighbourhood which she felt better reflected her heritage than her own neighbourhood: "It's very White, borderline racist [in my neighbourhood]. So, I'm in the house all the time, I don't ask friends, I'm not part of any community there or, I just basically live there." For Raquela, experiences of racism actively prevented her from building connections and accessing support where she lived. She spoke of not feeling part of the community and of staying in her home, and longing to move elsewhere after the pandemic (see Chapter 5). Therefore, what may be experienced as a landscape of care for some will be experienced as a space of anxiety, or exclusion, for others.

Among the South Asian respondents, relationships with neighbours tended to be organised around the exchange of food on special days, such as religious festivals, something that was greatly affected by social distancing rules. According to Aakaar, a 54-year-old Bangladeshi man: "The neighbourhood does not mix much but the relationship is cordial. We exchange food when it is Ramadan." This connection with neighbours through food exchange was meaningful even if it was restricted to special occasions. The impact of the pandemic on neighbourhood relationships was highlighted by Yasmin, a 64-year-old Pakistani woman: "It's not like before because we have a trend in our culture to exchange food but now, we don't see each other. We are scared to meet each other outside because we feel like maybe they can get [the] virus from us or we can get it from them."

For some participants who were isolated before the pandemic, being involved in a 'support bubble' cemented their relationships with neighbours, as with Patty, a 64-year-old White British woman living on her own, who suffered from severe depression and had very restricted physical mobility. Patty was estranged from her son and wider family so connections with neighbours were vital for her mental well-being: "The neighbour is allowed to come in and we sit, and we chat, and sometimes watch a film together." Prior to lockdown, Patty was active within her neighbourhood but after she began shielding, her day was focused around spending time on an arts and crafts pack sent by her local community centre:

'The way I live is each day as it comes and depending on how I'm feeling that day depends on what I do. And because the depression side of it has kicked in again, I'm not really doing much craftwork. Normally and at the beginning of the lockdown, I was doing a lot of craftwork … the one thing I am able to do and that is colouring but I do it on my mobile and my iPad. And that's what I spend my time doing at the moment is just colouring in, painting pictures using those apps. So in a way, I am keeping my brain busy.'

The arts and crafts packs were one way in which Patty could sustain her relationship with her wider neighbourhood network, one which had been ruptured through the requirement to shield. The pandemic opened people to new ways of renegotiating relationships and new occasions for neighbours to relate to each other, but there were also cases where this renegotiation was not possible, where experiences such as racism hindered the possibilities of developing meaningful connections. These different experiences illustrate some of the inequalities faced by our participants during lockdown. The imposition of social distancing also prompted people to explore new spaces where relationships could develop. Among our interviewees, this was particularly salient in the ways they engaged with nature and outdoor spaces.

Use of outdoor and communal spaces

The first lockdown in spring 2020 was characterised by long periods of warm weather which provided some relief from the constraints of being 'trapped' indoors. Being able to go outdoors was considered to be of great importance for many of the participants (see also Fancourt et al, 2022). Chris, a 66-year-old White British man, felt that: "We were very fortunate generally across the country that the first two or three months, the weather was very good." This view was confirmed by Amlika, a 62-year-old Bangladeshi woman: "The weather has been good so I have spent a lot of time in my own garden."

With social distancing guidelines prohibiting people from visiting friends and family in the home, doorsteps, driveways and gardens became important places for dropping off food deliveries or checking in on loved ones. Private gardens also became important spaces where some of our participants were able to continue to socialise with their families and friends while observing social distancing rules. Grace, a 72-year-old White British woman, described a visit from her daughter and son-in-law:

> 'They came up but we were all in the garden. They didn't come in the house and we socialised with social distance anyway. The garden is big enough to sit on one side or the other you know and my daughter's partner he did a couple of jobs for me.'

As social distancing restrictions eased, some activities were adapted so people could meet outdoors. Carl, a 65-year-old White British man, felt very isolated in the first interview, but was more optimistic when he was interviewed seven weeks later. He explained how the LGBTQ+ network he is part of had restarted their in-person meetings outdoors:

> 'We have had two meetings but we decided to have them, well we could only have them outside because of the virus so we had one in the park and about 20 people came. On that day it was 30 degrees, it was really hot but we sat in the shade like in little groups, you know close to each other but keeping a social distance and it just felt really, really good.'

However, not everyone had the advantage of access to outdoor space. Some participants who lived in sheltered accommodation talked about tensions

Figure 6.3: Grandparents in park

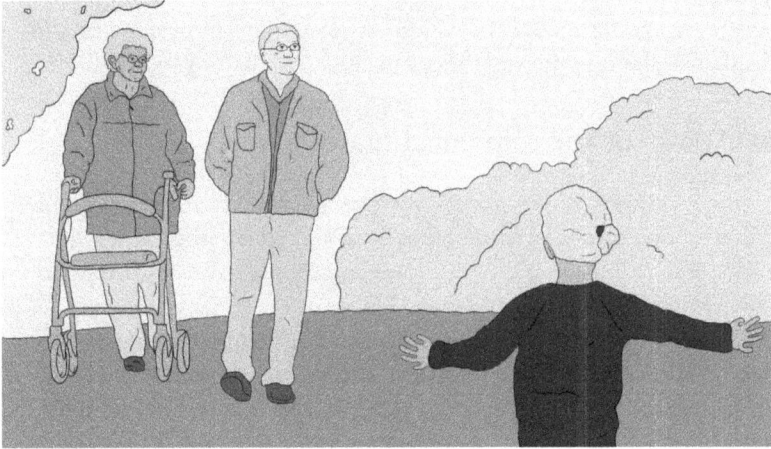

Figure 6.4: Out in the city

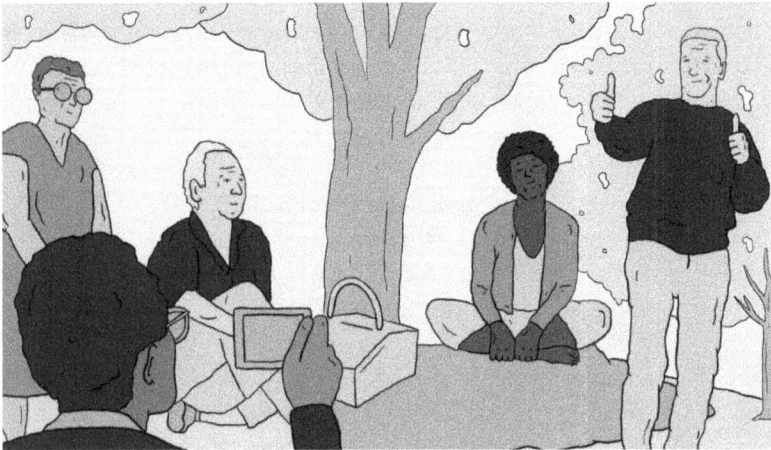

arising from restricted access to communal gardens due to social distancing rules. Irene, an 85-year-old White British woman living on her own in sheltered accommodation, described in her first interview how she enjoyed playing "Glenn Miller and all the old singers" on her patio and spoke to her neighbours from a distance. However, by the second interview, regulations had become much stricter and she could no longer use the communal garden in the same way. After her closest friend and neighbour contracted COVID-19, the residents were told by management to abstain from any form of social interaction. Irene was particularly distressed about how she was also banned from visiting her close friend in hospital:

'Because I'm on complete shutdown I'm having no visitors, the only people I'm speaking to is by phone. … No one is allowed in unless it's a medical thing and you have a carer coming, no it's complete isolation. … At the present time I'm not eating very much, I'm losing my appetite as well, it's not the same is it when you're not seeing anyone?'

George, who lived alone in sheltered housing, also experienced social distancing restrictions impacting on his relationship to his neighbours, which became more distant: "Before, I used to see two or three when we used to take the washing in on a Saturday to a laundrette. Now it's just that we're all separate, we don't see nobody else in there."

For respondents living in sheltered accommodation, the perception of home, which in some cases was only one bedroom went beyond the boundaries of the individual household, and also included communal gardens and laundry spaces. Irene's and George's examples shed light on the effect of unequal access to outdoor and communal spaces during the pandemic, in their cases resulting from additional regulations affecting their housing schemes, which added to their experience of isolation. It was also evident from accounts by Patty, Irene and George, who all lived on their own and had a restricted family network, that relationships with their neighbours often had a 'kin-like' quality. However, because of rules for tenants it was not straightforward to constitute a 'bubble' with a neighbour, an example of how older people living in such spaces at times found themselves in a 'double lockdown' (Buffel et al, 2021), where the consequences from the more general restriction of social distance were compounded by a lockdown within the home environment.

Figure 6.5: Alone in the laundry

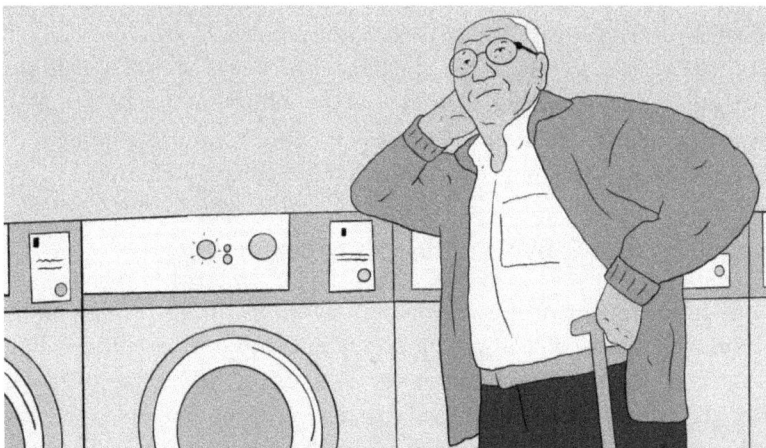

For many of those who were able to spend time outdoors, an increased interest in nature and wildlife was expressed. Dharti, a 50-year-old Sri Lankan woman, felt that she had

'become more interested in birdwatching. I have been looking at birds, you know we have a few bird feeders, so there are lots of birds coming to our garden. And I try to find out which type of birds who are coming and [I am] more and more interested about birds now.'

For some participants, access to a garden was important in reducing feelings of isolation. When asked whether she felt more isolated during the third lockdown. Miranda, an 84-year-old Black Caribbean woman living on her own, replied:

'Sometimes if I'm outside I can see them outside in their backyard and then we talk over the fence or across the fence I should say. Other people have [felt more isolated] but not for me. Because I can sort of, you know, find things to do and I can go out in the garden.'

For those participants who were advised to shield, gardens offered a precious space to relax. For example, Paula, a 75-year-old White British woman who identified as gay, had hardly seen anyone since March as her partner had been diagnosed with cancer just before the start of the lockdown. Gardening was the one activity that offered them both pleasure: "She [Paula's partner] does really well with the garden, and I like the garden, and she's been ordering all the plants and all the compost and all that, and they've been delivering it. So, we've been able to manage to do that."

Such comments highlight the benefits associated with green spaces during the pandemic when outdoor areas were seen as extensions of people's homes and where people could socialise at a distance, but we also identified inequality of access to such spaces, compounded by the pandemic. As with other areas of everyday life, the pandemic made people see old spaces and engage with old activities in new ways, while simultaneously making underlying inequalities more apparent. The observation also applied to the role of technology in the lives of older people during lockdown.

Reinventing relationships: the role of technology

An important feature of life under COVID-19 was the use of technology, notably as a means of combating social isolation and exclusion. Digital exclusion is especially relevant in the context of GM where Office for National Statistics data (2021) showed that 57 per cent of people aged 75 and over had not used the internet in the past three months or had never used the internet. Research by Hall et al (2022) in GM found that the COVID-19 pandemic did not seem to have led to substantially higher numbers of older people getting online, with increased use coming from those who were already using digital technology in various forms.

Our participants were fairly evenly divided at the first interview between 58 regular users pre-COVID-19, and 44 occasional or non-users. We found wide variations in how technology was used, with three main categories evident: regular users (computers, tablets and/or smart phones); occasional users; and non-users (digitally excluded and/or resistant to technology). The third interview with our participants revealed that being digitally connected had offered for many a crucial means of maintaining social connections. By the same token, 'digital exclusion' could be a significant barrier to maintaining relationships, with the majority of those mentioning 'feeling worse' or more 'depressed' lacking access to different kinds of technology and social media. The main themes identified by our participants regarding use of technology can be summarised as follows: keeping connections with family and friends who live locally and overseas; maintaining religious practice through technology; digital exclusion and fatigue; and connectivity within the LGBTQ+ community.

Keeping connected

Using technology to connect with family and friends was particularly important for special occasions, such as Ramadan, birthdays, anniversaries and funerals. For the South Asian participants, not being able to celebrate Ramadan with their extended family was a considerable challenge, but one mitigated though remote connections, as reported by Idris, a 56-year-old Bangladeshi woman:

'I have mainly been at home and focusing more on my spiritual well-being during the lockdown. I spent time with my grandchildren, watched heritage TV and connect[ed] via Zoom during Ramadan with the family. ... I can text messages via mobile to my friends or have conversations with my GP. I found connecting via Zoom kept me going as well as build my confidence of using digital systems.'

A number of our respondents were taught by younger members of their family, demonstrating how digital technology acted as an intergenerational medium that could enhance relationships. Andrea, an 80-year-old African Caribbean woman, reported: "My niece she's a bit more enlightened about the computer. So, when I have some problem with that, I will note them down and when she comes round I just tell her, please show me how to do this." Saamita, a 60-year-old Bangladeshi woman, said: "I use the telephone and also my grandkids help me to connect with other relatives on Zoom." And Farida commented that: "Before the pandemic I had never used Zoom or WhatsApp but my children have taught me, or do it for me, so everything is fine."

Doris, an 86-year-old White British woman, summarised the intergenerational help she received as follows:

> 'She [granddaughter] came round about a month ago, into the back garden ... so I'd sit on the patio, she'd be down through the garden at the bottom, and talk me through Zoom; the next morning, through my letterbox arrived a step-by-step four-page, step by step detail of how I access Zoom ... that's something I would never have done before.'

But what was perhaps the most striking discovery for those who started to use technology was how they could maintain different kinds of social connections. For Chaminda, a 60-year-old Sri Lankan man:

> 'It is hard, but luckily people have social media for example to deal with the loneliness difficulty. With social media you can connect with others, and it doesn't feel like you are lonely all day. Although you are at home, with modern technology you are not really at home. You can be with anybody that you want, and it is a way to cope with these difficulties.'

And Chika, a 51-year-old Black British woman, conveys a real sense of excitement about the possibilities of technology:

> 'I think in a way I feel that Covid has even made us get more contact with people. Well, I mean not physical contact, but with having a lot of days meetings and all that online, you can physically jump from one meeting to the other, which was not there, which you couldn't have done physically. You could have a meeting in Bolton, another meeting somewhere, you know, ten miles away, or five miles.'

Maintaining religious practice

For some, their online networks expanded across international boundaries. This was most clearly demonstrated by the ways in which some of our participants engaged with online faith networks. For example, Leroy, an 84-year-old Black British man originally from Barbados, had been a pastor for a number of years, but access to Zoom had greatly expanded his network. During the pandemic, he delivered teachings to people in Jamaica, Barbados, the United States and Canada, as well as in the UK.

Cameron, a 56-year-old African Caribbean man working as a nurse, was a member of a charismatic church. At the beginning of the lockdown in March, he and his family started attending services on Zoom. While collective singing with the congregation was no longer possible due to technological limitations, he and his family sang along with the preacher with their microphones on mute:

> 'I miss going to church but on the other hand I also have to follow the precautions and also make sure that I'm safe, my family are safe. The church is there all the time. We can go to church at any time. If everything is OK and we're not under restriction. We go to church at our own risk now. For now, I would say I will be on the Zoom.'

Joseph, a 69-year-old White British man living on his own who was a Jehovah's Witness, missed "the friendship" and his "brothers and sisters".

Figure 6.6: Cross-border technology

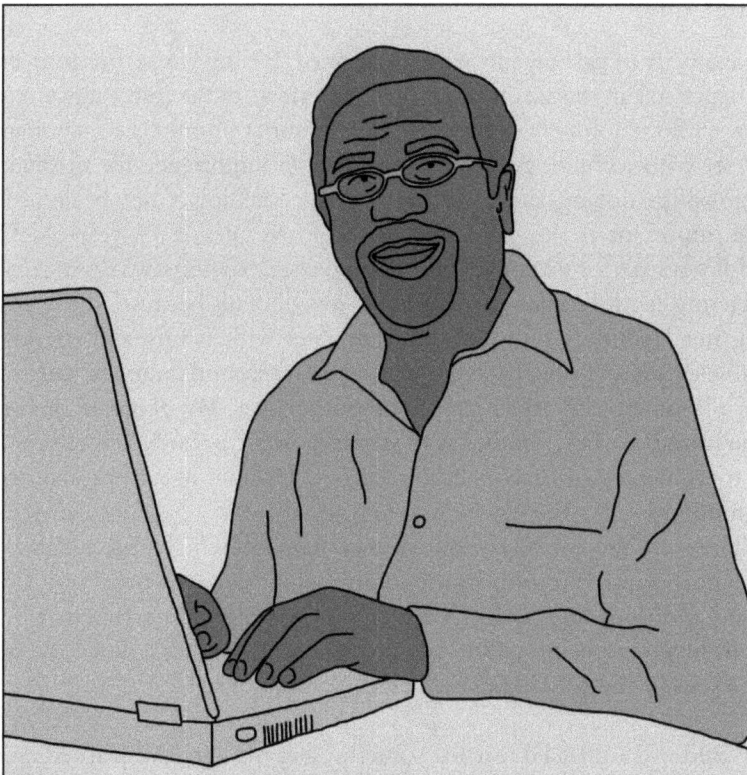

For Joseph, his congregation were like kin, so he learned to use Zoom in order to keep the connection with his "spiritual family":

'We just carry on as we would as if we were meeting together in our Kingdom Halls. At our Zoom meetings some of us sing along ... it's not as nice as meeting in public when we go to our Kingdom Halls but at least we can still have an interchange and ...hear talks from different Brothers.'

However, despite the benefits of Zoom, many participants, like Cameron and Joseph, missed the face-to-face dimension of religious practice. Some mentioned that 'there's no fellowship with people' because social interactions had disappeared. Rushnik, a 74-year-old Indian man, felt that he "would have benefited from religious gatherings; I think that would have helped. I tried Zoom church but it's not the same". And Kamal, a 61-year-old Indian man, said that he would "like to visit my mosque daily at least once a day and meet many friends and neighbours there, but with this lockdown it is difficult".

Digital exclusion

The majority of participants who mentioned 'feeling worse' or more 'down and depressed' in the second and third interviews of the research were often those without access to computers and/or smart phones. Engagement (or lack of) with technology was of considerable importance for maintaining relationships during the early part of the lockdown but became even more important as the pandemic wore on. Monica, a 76-year-old Black British woman, for example, did not own a smart phone which meant that contacting family members in Jamaica was difficult because of the cost of using her landline. With dwindling contact with family and friends she became even more isolated, commenting in her second interview that: "[My sons] phone me and come round when they can. My grandchildren can't come round. ... Everybody has to stay in now ... nobody can visit ... you feel more depressed than anything else. ... I would like to be able to use a computer."

There were also a smaller number of participants who had access and skills for digital communication but reported being 'sick and tired' of it by the second and third interview. Doris, an 86-year-old White British woman, told us how embracing online technology had given her a new lease of life at the start of the pandemic:

'I kind of say that I'd learned something at my age, I've learned, and realised how stupid it was to have this block about not having the internet, because it's opened another way for me to communicate with people, and another way to attend meetings. I never would have thought that possible, so that's a good part of being locked in the house.'

However, interviewed six months later, she had become less enthusiastic:

'I did start going on the Zoom meetings but then they stressed me out that much that I thought, well I sat down, and I thought I'm either losing my mind or I'm stressed and identified that I was stressed and then what was stressing me was the thought of the Zoom, so I stopped.'

Technology also offered little substitute for being physically present with family members, especially during difficult times. Yasmin, a 64-year-old Pakistani woman, explained the pain of not being able to be close to her mother during her final days, telling our researchers that "the regret is going to be with me forever". The impact of restrictions prohibited families from being together during their loved one's final days and to mark their passing was shared by many other participants. Not being able to comfort other family members by visiting them in person was particularly hard. "I feel really bad about it", Gatik, a 59-year-old Bangladeshi man, said. "[I]t shouldn't be like this."

Technology and the LGBTQ+ community

Participants from the LGBTQ+ community demonstrated some of the most highly skilled and sustained engagement with technology. Due to past experiences of being criminalised because of their sexual orientation, members of the LGBTQ+ group were especially affected by the closure of places to meet. With a history of social exclusion, the LGBTQ+ community relied on safe spaces where they could meet and maintain supportive relationships. These types of 'kin-like' relations with other members of the LGBTQ+ community were vital for those who were not in regular contact with their families or who did not have children (Weeks et al, 2001). Samantha, for example, is a 69-year-old White British woman in a same-sex relationship with no children. Both Samantha and her wife are also only children. During lockdown they witnessed many of their neighbours relying on children to do shopping and run errands:

'Because of the nature of how things were, women of our age that are lesbians, tend to not have children. If you don't have children, you don't have grandchildren and you will see the absences that flow out from that. Also, as it happens, we are both only children, so no brothers, no sisters, no nieces, no nephews.'

Samantha's landscape of care was constituted by her community of identity rather than her family, and technology was key in terms of maintaining her support network. She was also very much aware that giving care to others helped her cope with the lockdown: "I'm still doing my online counselling, so I'm doing a service you know looking outside of myself. ... I think that's the key thing is, I've got connection, I've got an outward-looking thing in my life. I've got the counselling clients."

Many groups and activities moved online during the pandemic and our participants showed increasing proficiency over the three interviews in adapting to virtual social life, even if actual human contact was often deeply missed. Brian, a 74-year-old White British man who identified as gay, attended an online wine party, "where we've all opened a bottle of wine in our own houses, and all chat over Zoom"; and Douglas, a 70-year-old man who lived alone, created a weekly podcast where he told the story of his life through music. He also removed furniture from his living room to join his line-dance classes remotely and by his third interview, Douglas had become used to having dance classes on Zoom: "The guys who run it have done a fantastic job in keeping the group together. We do dancing. We chat in between dances. They tell us any news. So, it's a great form of interaction, keeping in touch with people."

Carl, a 70-year-old White British man, started to spend more time producing podcasts for an older people's radio station. While Suzanne, a 72-year-old White British woman, got involved with an older people's collective where she explored her creative potential:

> 'I'm involved with Talking About My Generation, we made a video, which I recorded ... if I can support other people, that gives me pleasure, and also, it's a two-way street with chit chat. It's not, you know, it's not me listening, it's not them just rabbiting away and me listening. It's a two-way thing, because they're my friends.'

Suzanne also described some of the online activities she had attended during Manchester Pride: "Pride in Ageing with all kinds of things there, I was on a quiz during, an absolutely crazy quiz during Virtual Manchester Pride where there were three drag queens setting the questions, and a bunch of us oldies, LGBTers giving the answers."

Relationships within the LGBTQ+ community were reciprocal. Both giving and receiving care and support were highly valued by our participants. The experience of changing relationships during the pandemic demonstrate the long-term effects of stigma and discrimination and how these experiences continued to shape the landscapes of care of which people were part of. Being cut off from family or feeling alienated from neighbourhoods was not necessarily a new experience for many of our LGBTQ+ participants.

But although there were challenges, many of these participants were able to continue connections within their community with relative ease, using online spaces. Therefore, despite the fact they were operating at a physical distance, there were examples of emotional closeness and the expansion of social networks. This is a reminder that care can be both a physical and emotional labour (Conradson, 2003), and that in the context of social distancing, emotional labour was paramount.

The pandemic has highlighted the importance of digital technology as a coping mechanism for older adults. Among those who were shielding, online connectivity proved to be invaluable in maintaining social connections of various kinds. It enabled people to pursue social activities, to connect with family members, to purchase goods and services, and to receive much-needed emotional support. In some cases, technology allowed people to expand their landscapes of care at a time when physical proximity was heavily restricted. However, it is certainly the case that for those detached from online communication, life was considerably restricted during the lockdowns, with the possibility of them falling further behind as digital communication becomes a more important part of everyday life.

Conclusion

The pandemic had multiple and complex implications for older people's relationships in our study. The examples discussed in this chapter provide important insights into how the landscapes of care that had provided some with a degree of protection from social isolation before the pandemic were significantly challenged during the successive periods of lockdown. There were examples of relationships becoming more distant, and some becoming closer; some participants developed new networks of support with new spaces of care emerging as a result. There were, therefore, complex and uneven patterns of change that emerged from our interviews across the 12-month period, changes that can be characterised as both a *contraction and expansion of social relationships* and a *reconfiguration of landscapes of care*.

Some participants felt their social worlds had *contracted* and become centred on the home as other social spaces and networks became more *restricted*. Landscapes of care within the home became tense sites of renegotiation of caring roles, as well as spaces for reconnection and appreciation. Landscapes of care beyond the home were also reorientated and different spatial patterns of care emerged. The understanding of home extended to spaces outside the dwelling. Virtual space and public outdoor settings all took on new meanings within an extended landscape of care. Neighbourhoods also took on new significance, as sources of care and support for some, while being sites of hostility and alienation for others. As important spaces of care became closed off to older people, new spaces of care emerged and took on new meaning within the home and garden, as well as in public and virtual spaces. For some participants, landscapes of care increased beyond international boundaries, while for others they became vanishingly small. Some of these new landscapes of care relied on existing networks, as in the case of faith groups, but they also exposed the inequalities related to digital exclusion, anxieties about going out, and the isolation experienced by those without access to outdoor spaces.

Social distancing reconfigured the landscapes of care for older people interviewed in this study. The government's rules required people to remain physically distant in order to both care for and care about others, which caused the need to rethink our understanding of both physical and emotional proximity and distance within caring relationships. The participants responded to this in different ways and their capacity to renegotiate the spatial arrangement of their relationships was unequal. This chapter has demonstrated how access to, and ability to engage with, both virtual and outdoor spaces was key in enabling older people to maintain caring relationships. However, this was not always a question of individual capacity but structural inequality and this study has made evident that care and support were unevenly experienced before the pandemic. To add to this, those older people who had experienced social exclusion and discrimination *before* the pandemic were often further disadvantaged as a result of COVID-19 (see, further, Buffel et al, 2021). Our findings also highlight that differences in the use of technology can mean new forms of *inequality* within the older population. In summary, some relationships adapted while others flourished, but overall, relationships became more limited in a variety of ways.

7

The role of community organisations and social infrastructure

Introduction

Chapter 6 examined how the pandemic created added pressures to the support received by some of the individuals and groups interviewed for our research. An important response came from organisations and individuals within communities themselves, with what is known as the Voluntary, Community and Social Enterprise (VCSE) sector playing a significant role in the landscapes of care for groups such as older people. This chapter discusses the experience of a range of VCSE organisations across GM, looking at the challenges posed by social distancing and the demand for new ways of working within communities.

The chapter draws on longitudinal interviews with 21 community leaders, organisers and activists working and volunteering in organisations supporting older people as well as people working in local government. The discussion examines the role they played in responding to the pandemic and how this changed over time. As outlined in Chapter 3, organisations were drawn from across the voluntary sector in GM, including those working in particular neighbourhoods, charities focused on older people such as local branches of Age UK, equalities organisations such as the Manchester BME Network and the LGBT Foundation, and groups working with particular ethnic minority communities such as the KYP, the Ethnic Health Forum and the Caribbean and African Health Network (CAHN). Also included in this chapter are interviews with those in local government involved in the delivery of policy and practice to support older people in communities, as well as individuals involved in more informal community activity to support older people. A full list of the organisations can be found in Table 3.1.

The sample of organisations reflects the diversity of cross-sector approaches to ageing policy which have developed in GM over many decades. Although the wider network is strong, as evidenced through GM's status as a World Health Organization age-friendly region, organisations and groups within the network vary in size and resources. This means that they came into the pandemic with varying capacities to respond to the needs of the groups and individuals with whom they worked.

Following the longitudinal design of the research, the chapter is structured to present the evolving experience of the community and voluntary sector throughout the first year of the pandemic. The discussion explores the actions taken by organisations in the initial weeks and months, and then examines how services were adapted and reinvented over a 12-month period, in response to changing circumstances and needs among older people and the neighbourhoods in which they lived. The chapter also considers the impact of the services developed or maintained, both on older people as users and as people directly involved in their design and delivery. To conclude, the discussion considers the future needs of the sector in continuing to support older people.

Initial responses to the pandemic

The early weeks of the lockdown provided a number of challenges for the organisations interviewed. The initial stages of the pandemic were described as forming part of an 'emergency response', where organisations reacted to the issues in hand before moving on to a more strategic style of planning later in the year. One community organiser commented that "these have been extraordinary times with a lot of ... firefighting". Karen, a staff member from Age UK Salford, spoke for many with her comment on the early phase of the pandemic:

'For six or eight weeks we [staff and volunteers] didn't see much of each other. It was all hands on deck within our organisation, [access to] food was the priority. Reflecting on what we could do with staff in a safe way. It took a long time to sort out the practicalities. We pulled staff out of the hospital café and services were closed. Phone calls had to be reorganised because of the increasing number of people calling. Lockdown started on 23rd March. The previous Thursday the risk assessment started.'

Staff and volunteer shortages were high, due to people being ill with the virus or having to shield or self-isolate, which meant capacity was stretched from the outset. Some organisations lost staff through the operation of the furlough scheme. The most immediate change was the switch to home-working as offices and community centres were forced to close. This shift was disruptive for everyone, but for some of the smaller organisations limited access to personal laptops and mobile telephones presented additional barriers, as described by Atfat, a project officer from the Ethnic Health Forum:

'We were able to apply for a grant from Manchester City Council to get a laptop and mobile phone for staff so they could continue to work from home. Even then this is taking some adjustment as everyone is getting to grips with new ways of working on things such as Zoom so there have been some challenges around training for staff and some need more support than others.'

Even with the appropriate equipment, many staff faced combining home-working while juggling other caring and home-schooling responsibilities. Organisations were able to use their existing relationships in the community to contact those whom they thought might need assistance. These initial contacts, often made around the provision of food and medicines, were also used as more general welfare checks. Those interviewed described how they were able to refer people to other organisations if needed, as well as ensuring the people to whom they spoke had contact details in case of emergencies. Initial contacts were generally made via telephone and social media, word of mouth, and referrals from other community hubs and service providers to identify and reach older people who were unknown to organisations. However, there were concerns that the closure of many public spaces meant that certain individuals would be missed, as Sally from Age UK Wigan explained:

'There is always going to be people we aren't able to reach because people aren't gathering in the places like they used to, like libraries and doctor's surgeries etc. We would like to be able to mail [an information newsletter] to the whole borough but we can't because we don't have the funds for that.'

Some of the services developed also required online staff training to meet social distancing guidelines. A large number of organisations relied upon volunteers, themselves often aged 70 and over but now required to shield. Within weeks, or days in some cases, organisations had to develop a new range of activities to cater for people unable to leave their home and who had no means of engaging remotely. One organisation described how they phoned over 1,000 people who were registered with them to tell them about the changes being implemented.

The early months of the pandemic represented, then, a period of significant disruption for the community and voluntary sector. However, as described in the following section, almost immediately organisations started to implement changes to their ways of working so that they were able to continue existing services and provide new ones to meet the emerging demands of the pandemic.

Adaptations to services and support

In this section four main adaptations to services and support for older people are discussed, which emerged as key areas of concern for the various

Figure 7.1: Closed community centre

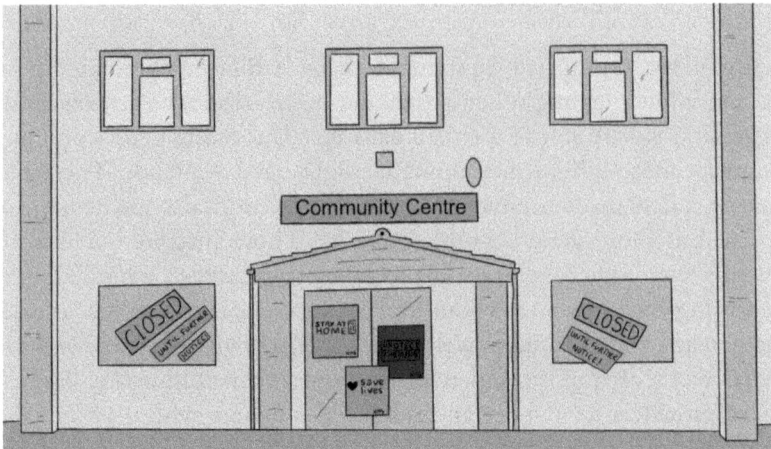

interviewees: *provision and distribution of food*; *moving services online*; *telephone befriending services and other ways of keeping in touch*; and *the provision of mental health and well-being services*.

Provision and distribution of food

The provision and distribution of food, which formed a significant part of the work carried out by community organisations during the pandemic, took several forms and responded to different types of needs. In some cases, it involved collecting and delivering food for those unable to leave their homes and who had no one else to help them. In other instances, it entailed providing free or subsidised food to households who were struggling financially. Services such as food banks and emergency food parcels were often provided free or, in the case of the delivery of cooked meals, with a small charge to recipients. One organisation commented that they began charging a small fee for their food provision service after feedback that this fostered a degree of self-respect for the beneficiaries. Other organisations worked with local community hubs to provide culturally appropriate food to older community members.

The KYP, a community organisation in Rochdale, working with members of the Kashmiri and Pakistani communities, found that food parcels provided by the local authority, as part of the emergency response to the pandemic, did not always cater for the needs of South Asian families. According to one of the organisers at the KYP:

'The local community hubs were offering emergency food parcels to older people but they only had two options, vegetarian or non-vegetarian, no other dietary requirements were considered. Many South Asian households opted for non-vegetarian but weren't able to eat a lot of what was sent to them because the meat was not Halal.'

In response, the KYP started collecting and distributing their own food donations to ensure that older people had access to culturally appropriate and Halal provisions. In the first stages of the pandemic, the organisation reported distributing over 750 food parcels to local households. When the KYP were interviewed for the second time, in the autumn of 2020, the provision of food had become one of their main activities and they had set up a food pantry to collect and store donations. Shenaz commented that they had seen rising rates of poverty in the area and, as a result, saw this development as a permanent feature of the KYP's work:

'There is going to be a longer-term need. We feel that poverty has increased in the area and that the local emergency food support that was set up at the start of the pandemic is starting to fade away. With more and more families being financially impacted by the pandemic … the ability of families to support their older relatives is being put under pressure, so we see this is a longer-term need.'

Moving services and activities online

Moving a variety of support services online was a feature of work across GM. Activities and groups that had previously been delivered face-to-face, such as social groups, chair-based exercise sessions and well-being classes, were transferred to online platforms such as Zoom. As the pandemic continued, the use of online platforms developed further, with some organisations adding a range of electronic games, as well as repurposing funds to send members items through the post, such as craft packs to support some of their online activities.

For many older people, the pandemic was the first time they felt they needed to engage with others using online platforms. Therefore, organisations provided additional support to enable their members to become more confident in accessing online technology. For example, Levenshulme Good Neighbours offered a befriending service and IT coaching on how to use hardware, software and social media. 'Tech and Tea at Home' was another initiative to encourage digital inclusion run by Inspiring Communities Together, based in Salford. This programme organised volunteers to visit people on their doorstep to provide guidance on how to use their computer. Those who used the service were then invited to online sessions in getting more proficient in IT, in some cases, using tablets supplied by the programme at a subsidised rate. Subsequent online sessions then looked at issues around healthy eating, keeping entertained and staying safe online.

Initiatives such as 'Tech and Tea' were labour-intensive but had largely positive and sometimes unexpected results, including attracting new service users. For example, one organiser was surprised by the number of men who had joined their online group, as in her experience men were often more difficult to engage in organised group activities: "Normally there would be more women, but Covid changed that, perhaps because it's just a matter of turning the computer on, maybe their wife joined and they are in the same room so they join too. We had a 'sporting memories' initiative, so that attracted men as well.'

Online activities were also felt to be a way of providing opportunities for social interaction within existing social networks. One community organisation noted how Zoom fostered a new type of intimacy, as people felt more at ease talking to organisations from the comfort of their own home. In some instances, moving services online was not regarded as feasible, either because those involved were unable to access online technologies or because the nature of the service meant communicating online was not felt to be appropriate. For example, in the case of services dealing with confidential and sensitive material, the Ethnic Health Forum found that their information and advice service worked better for older people over the telephone and using WhatsApp:

'If a client wants help translating a letter or filling in a form they are able to take a photo of the documentation and send it via WhatsApp to a member of staff but then for staff to talk them through how to complete the form over the phone is difficult. Although some people are happy using smart phones for messages and social media, downloading a form from their emails is a different matter.'

Issues surrounding digital exclusion, whether through access to technologies or lack of confidence in their use, were challenging for organisations to face in their efforts to adapt services during the pandemic. Some were cautious about moving all of their meetings and activities online too quickly and consequently excluding some individuals. Daniel who worked for the LGBT Foundation was conscious of not leaving anyone behind because of digital exclusion:

'About a third of people on the Advisory group are able to use Zoom and happy to do so, another third either don't have access to the technology or are opposed to using it feeling that it is not a substitute for meeting face-to-face. The final third are somewhere in the middle: they are willing to use the technology but may need some support in doing so.'

Some organisations were able to attract new service users through online platforms, and for older people, there was the benefit of maintaining social contacts and developing new skills in using digital technology. However, transferring services was not without challenges. Significant resources were required to help people to become digitally connected, and in some cases, digital exclusion meant alternative mediums of connecting were needed, as reviewed in the next section of this chapter.

Telephone befriending and other ways of keeping in touch

Considerable time and effort was reported by organisations in maintaining connections with older people who were either already socially isolated, or at risk of becoming further isolated, due to the pandemic. Where people were unable to participate in online activities, alternative methods of communication and staying in touch were used. By far the most important was the telephone, which was seen by some stakeholders as more inclusive, as most older people had access to a landline. Almost all the organisations expanded their telephone befriending services, and also carried out welfare checks by telephone. As one organiser commented: "Our starting point was the phone conversation. For some people that weekly telephone call is their main social interaction." These calls helped to find out if people needed any additional support. At the same time, they also provided a chance to have an informal chat for those who might otherwise have been at increased risk of social isolation. Telephone calls provided a lifeline, especially for service users who were struggling with having limited social contacts.

As well as the risks of social isolation, and the need for information, some organisations developed telephone befriending schemes which helped continue a sense of community and belonging among particular groups of people. For example, the LGBT Foundation set up the 'Rainbow Brew

Figure 7.2: Telephone befriending

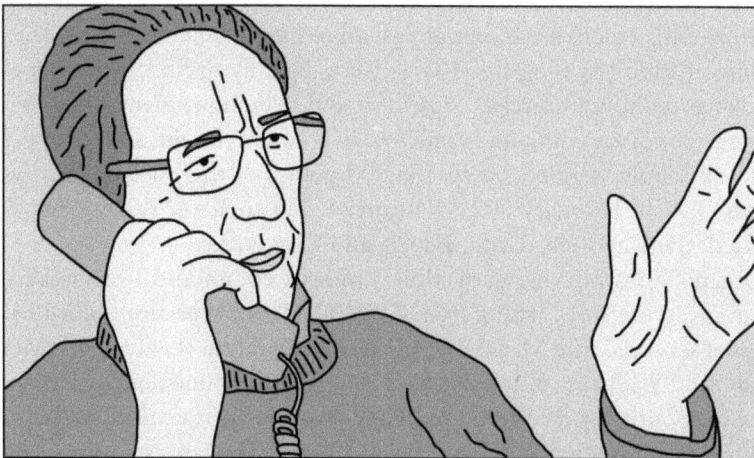

Buddies' telephone befriending service, in response to people from the LGBTQ+ community experiencing increased isolation during the lockdown. The service paired up users with volunteers to have a regular telephone catch-up for the length of time it takes to drink a cup of tea or coffee.

A similar support role was found in the use of WhatsApp groups to disseminate information to large numbers of people. This was the case with a WhatsApp group created by the KYP for the members of their Elders Group (most of whom were women), which was successful in keeping people in touch with one another and with the service. The online messaging group was used daily to share information about the service, health advice and regular updates on government restrictions. It also offered a forum for discussions, with many women providing peer-to-peer support and advice.

Mental health and well-being support

The challenges arising from social distancing, as well as existing pressures facing many living in poverty, meant that many organisations saw a steep increase in the need for mental health support for particular groups of older people. Mental health and well-being needs were addressed though a number of avenues. Due to the reluctance sometimes encountered when having conversations around mental health, organisations tended to address this issue from different angles, not all of which had an explicit focus on mental health. Examples include printed guides on maintaining health and well-being during the pandemic, initiatives to encourage people to stay active, as well as more interventionist approaches such as counselling and advice services.

In May 2020, the GM Ageing Hub (part of the Combined Authority) worked in collaboration with researchers at the University of Manchester to design and distribute a 'Keeping well at home' booklet for those aged 50 and over living in the GM area. The booklet, which was updated at the end of 2020 with a focus on 'Keeping well this winter', aimed to address the gap in information reaching those who were digitally excluded. It contained guidance on home exercises, nutrition and hydration, mental well-being, staying connected with others and how to access key health and other public and community services, with 136,000 copies of the booklet distributed across GM. In February 2021, a further 8,300 copies of the booklet were printed, translated into Urdu, Bangla and Easy Read.

Organisations working with ethnic minority communities recognised the need, given pressures arising from COVID-19, for specialist mental health support services. The Manchester BME Network was involved in a Mental Health and Wellbeing pilot project offering holistic counselling to individuals from the South Asian community. They organised private therapists to offer sessions about coping with anxiety and stress. The sessions were open to

Figure 7.3: Talking through glass

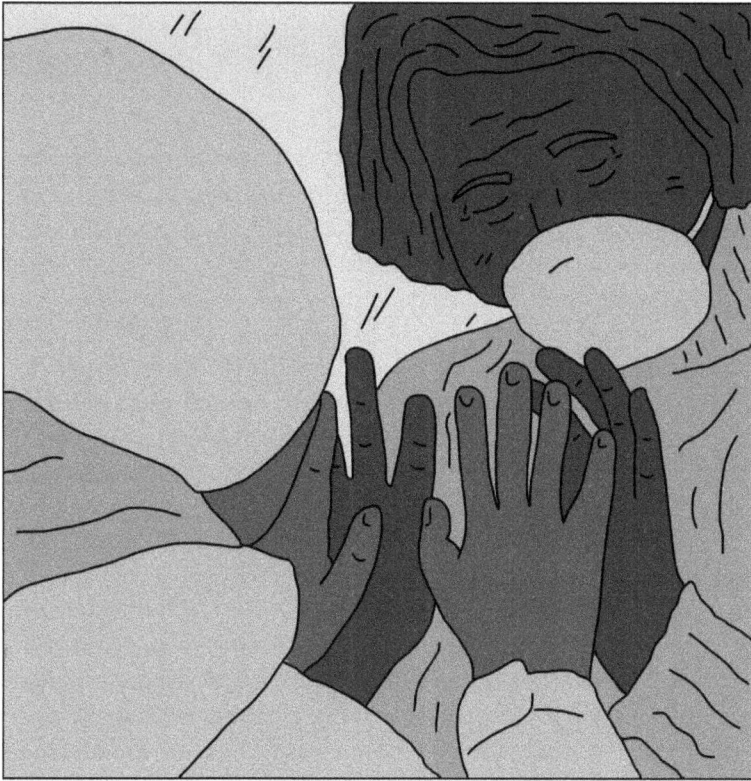

all ages, but many of those accessing the services were over-50s. Also, one interviewee commented that she had been surprised by the number of older men accessing the service, and that they recruited a male therapist in response to this demand.

The CAHN responded to a similar gap identified within the Black African and Caribbean community around bereavement counselling. It was felt that mainstream bereavement counselling services were ill-equipped to address the impact of the disruption to traditional ways of grieving that social distancing had caused. In response, the CAHN helped to set up a counselling service staffed by bereavement counsellors from within the community in response to this need.

Organisations with access to green spaces were able to run group and one-to-one activities, once restrictions began to lift in the summer of 2020. These spaces provided an important additional resource to encourage people to get outdoors and look after their physical and mental health. One community organiser explained:

'From July, the management of the allotment had to include sanitising of tools and outside toilets because a great number of people started to come to volunteer. It's been a life saver as the allotment helped combat social isolation. In addition, volunteers could take home a bag of fresh produce from the gardens.'

A similar initiative, 'Inspiring Communities Together', started to deliver a 'Walk and Talk' service, where a member of staff would accompany one or two older people for a walk around a local park. History walks were also added to this programme in an effort to appeal to people's different needs and interests, and a video was made to show how people could use the park safely and with confidence. The 'Rainbow Brew Buddies' also extended their befriending service, providing volunteers to accompany people one-to-one to go back to public spaces once they reopened, in an effort to build people's confidence around returning to activities and events.

The role of older people in networks of support

As seen in Chapter 6, many older people were themselves key actors in the landscapes of care that emerged within communities. One such example is Joyce, a woman in her 80s, who was an important figure within the age-friendly community in GM, as well as the African Caribbean community. She described how she started contacting some of the people she knew through the age-friendly network, in the early stages of the pandemic:

'Some friends had told me they might need a phone call as well and that's how I started phoning up members from the Greater Manchester age-friendly network and also from the age-friendly board, phoning them up and asking them, how are you doing? I think it was just a pleasure to listen to them talk and hear how they are coping.'

Joyce regularly telephoned seven or eight people, a role which she took on her own initiative, saying she "just felt like I needed to do this". Joyce is one example of many older people in this research who were part of informal networks of support, either in the neighbourhoods in which they lived or within their communities of identity or experience. As well as providing a friendly ear, these individuals also functioned as informal community connectors, where they were able to signpost and in some cases inform older people about services or support networks. Joyce described an example of a woman she knew called Janet who was supporting a neighbour called Denise:

'Janet is wonderful, she lives in Bury. I think Denise is in her 80s. She does a lot on her phone as well. Because somebody who was really in a dire situation … she was told about a lady who is in social isolation [shielding] and was very anxious because of [access to] food. So Janet gave her the number of the local authority and that was sorted out but not only that, Denise said she phoned up later on to find out if things had been sorted out. So she followed up.'

This excerpt demonstrates the vital role played by older people as key connectors in their communities, as well as the importance of the continued use of the telephone in maintaining connections during the pandemic.

Gaps in support for older people

During the second interview undertaken early in 2021, community organisers were asked about what they thought were *remaining gaps* in the support for older people. The main areas they identified included: *issues around mental health*; *lack of culturally relevant services*; *loss of opportunities for face-to-face contact*; and *digital exclusion*.

Supporting mental health and well-being

Many stakeholders commented on what they viewed as the deterioration of older people's mental health and well-being during the pandemic, confirming findings from older people discussed in previous chapters. Some organisers expressed concern about particular groups they supported who had "gone downhill really badly", and pointed to the need for enhanced emotional and mental health support. One remarked on the change in some people's emotional resilience to the lockdown as time went on, and how initial 'stoicism' had given way to less positive feelings, and darker questions being asked such as 'what's my life about?' Others commented that some older people had become 'hermit-like', and were feeling reluctant to go out of their homes (again, reinforced by observations in Chapter 6). While many organisations offered emotional support, either online or via telephone, the unprecedented circumstances of the pandemic and increased levels of need meant that in some cases, areas of concern were being missed. The skills and expertise available to meet high levels of need were unavailable in many instances, suggesting major concerns about the adequacy of mental health support given the long-term damage created by the pandemic.

The need for culturally relevant and accessible information and services

Early in the pandemic, many organisations working with ethnic minority communities felt that more effort should be made to provide information for those with lower levels of English literacy. An interviewee from the KYP gave the example of an information leaflet from the local authority about the local community hubs and emergency support available. An English-language version of the pamphlet was the only one available for a considerable period during the first wave of the pandemic. Local authorities made efforts to address the needs of BAME communities by, for example, translating information leaflets into different languages. However, one stakeholder from the South Asian community remarked that translation alone was not always sufficient, and that services needed to be complemented by culturally sensitive and accessible information. For example, it was noted that the image on the front of one information leaflet was of an older White woman, leaving the organiser to think that many people who did not identify with the image would have considered it irrelevant to their needs.

A similar sentiment was expressed by organisers regarding concerns within communities about vaccines for COVID-19. Several responded by hosting webinars involving medics from individual BAME communities to answer queries and discuss concerns. Once again, although many organisations did their best to respond to these gaps in accessible information, they felt more could have been done by statutory services, as in the following comment from Shenaz with the KYP:

'It all comes down to funding … support and engagement is only with the larger charities and the more arms-length sections of local authority, not with grass roots organisations and those working with marginalised communities such as ourselves. [Some people] tried to engage with statutory services for some help but were getting nowhere, ending up relying on voluntary organisations and neighbourhoods. … Some people have also been returning to their country of origin when they can. Not sure whether this is permanent or just for now as they feel they have more support there … in times of crisis and emergency when people are cut off from their usual support, many members of the South Asian community do not feel statutory services can meet their needs or they are not able to access their services.'

Loss of opportunities for face-to-face contact

Loss of access to physical spaces was highlighted by almost all organisers, when asked about the kind of facilities people were missing. This also confirms findings from our interviews with older people themselves, that online platforms were often a poor substitute for face-to-face interaction. The need for social interaction was a gap that many organisations were unable to address due to social distancing measures. Online interactions and keeping in touch via telephone calls and WhatsApp groups were vital lifelines for many. However, they did not replace face-to-face contact. Although some organisations did reintroduce some small group and one-to-one activities when regulations allowed, opportunities for casual drop-ins that had previously been offered were missing. This type of informal socialising, often unstructured and without any expectation or obligation, has long been a vital part of building social networks for many community organisations. Fears were expressed that losing this type of social contact would further isolate individuals who were less confident about attending more formal groups.

Digital exclusion and further isolation

Despite their best efforts, all of the organisations interviewed were concerned that some older people became further isolated by the pandemic due to digital exclusion. Lack of access, competence and desire to engage with online technologies made it difficult, if not impossible, to maintain contact with some older people. Due to the suspension or restriction of face-to-face services, stakeholders grew increasingly concerned that individuals and groups of older people who had been difficult to reach before the pandemic were now more at risk of 'slipping through the net' due to digital exclusion and increased risk of isolation. Outreach work, where organisations would attend different community spaces in order to engage with those who were not already coming to their services, had to be suspended during lockdown. Therefore, organisations had to rely on their existing knowledge of people in their communities and informal networks.

Existing support networks in the immediate neighbourhood protected some older people from social isolation in the early days of the pandemic. Our interviews with older people found multiple instances of support being provided by neighbours and family, filling gaps in services provided by statutory agencies. However, an organiser from the LGBT Foundation commented that some of the people they supported were hesitant to ask neighbours for help if they were not 'out' in their neighbourhoods. Equally, some LGBTQ+ older people were reported to be reluctant to get involved with volunteering in their local neighbourhoods due to concerns around stigma and discrimination.

Residents of sheltered accommodation were not completely protected from feeling isolated where they lived. Both organisers and participants in this study relayed stories of restricted access to communal areas, including gardens and laundry rooms, thus limiting opportunities for social contact (see Chapter 6). In one case, stakeholders related stories of residents feeling a lack of choice and consultation in the changes affecting their homes, with 'tape being put across communal areas and policing via CCTV'. Our research offered similar accounts of older people living in sheltered accommodation feeling as though they were not being treated as responsible adults.

Isolation and disengagement from services were not just concerns for the present, but for the future too, as many stakeholders voiced concerns about further disenfranchisement of some groups of older people from communities and service provision. One stakeholder within the South Asian community expressed her concern about access to primary care services all moving online and the impact this might have on older members of the community.

Working with socially excluded groups

Engaging with groups experiencing marginalisation and exclusion was an important challenge for community organisations. Factors that left people at risk of marginalisation varied considerably but organisations expressed concerns about groups with limited English and literacy, carers, people with complex health needs and those without children. However, through the interviews with organisations and volunteers, it became clear that many of their concerns were around people with complex and multiple needs who did not neatly fit into existing definitions of being at risk of social isolation.

Helen, a community activist living and working on a social housing estate, explained the challenges of maintaining contact through the pandemic with older people who were reluctant to engage with services:

'You have a group without family. Not good with technology. Not very good expressing emotions. Difficult to let people in. They don't want social services help. I have got all the trauma of helping people to get services but they still feel that government is something to be wary of because of their past when they worked on the side [paid in cash to avoid paying tax]. A lot of them don't access the usual kinds of support. And then the informal sources [of support] have gone.'

Helen's reflections highlight the multiple inequalities which affect some older people's lives. Martin, a volunteer in another neighbourhood, had similar concerns, particularly relating to residents he had been working with in organising a men's social group:

'I know Adam which was the person I was most concerned about … got himself a smart phone and I have been lending him books. He did not have a smart phone before and no internet access. He accessed [the internet] before via computers in the [public] library [free of charge] and the church. Last time I spoke to him he was trying to set the phone up. He lives in our [tower] block and he suffers from depression which isolates him anyway.'

Organisations and volunteers such as Helen and Martin have spent many years developing relationships of trust and understanding, working with isolated individuals, such as the single men referred to in these quotes, in order to try and break down some of the barriers preventing individuals from accessing help and support. There was a clear concern that the impact of the pandemic would undermine this work, as expressed by Martin: "We had a group of seven hard to reach people coming along to the meetings [prior to the pandemic]. Hopefully not all is lost. Hoping to run workshops at some point in the future in a socially responsible way."

As well as being able to reach people and maintain contact, organisations also expressed concern around meeting the specific needs of certain groups vulnerable to discrimination. For example, staff from the LGBT Foundation had concerns that much of the messaging from government around checking up on older family members at the start of the pandemic was heteronormative and did not take into account that many older LGBTQ+ adults might not have children or be estranged from them and their wider family networks. The messaging was felt to be alienating to the community, making it more difficult for people to ask for help, especially when there was such an emphasis in public discourse around neighbourhood level support. The Foundation was concerned that such a narrative overlooked the fact that some older people may not have had positive relationships with their neighbours.

More broadly, many organisations were anxious that despite their best efforts adapting services, not being able to host face-to-face activities was undermining their ability to reach out to marginalised groups. Kareem explained his concern about the effects of a closure of an important community space:

'People used to come to Inspire [a local community centre] for a coffee and this would take the whole morning. Now they have nothing to do. If they are on the phone it is only for ten minutes and what else do they do with their time? The social contact is missing.'

For organisations working with minority groups, the inability to meet in physical spaces was particularly acute. Staff from the LGBT Foundation reflected on the lack of opportunities during the pandemic for older LGBTQ+ adults to meet face-to-face with those who shared their identity and to be able to access inclusive spaces:

'For many people their LGBT identity hasn't been affirmed throughout the pandemic as people have been cut off from the groups and organisations where this is central. For example when people have been engaging with health care services they feel their identity is not recognised and also where people have reconnected with family due to checking up on them it has been the same. Therefore, people are really missing the spaces and opportunities to have their identity recognised.'

An additional concern was the pressure on organisations to meet the specific needs of different groups when faced with the death of a partner or relative. This was evident, for example, within the Muslim community where the loss of friends and relatives could not be marked with traditional Islamic customs. As community organiser Kareem explained:

'For a Muslim, when you leave this world, there are the last rites, but none of this could happen. People feel so guilty. I tried to call the family [of the deceased], but now they have stopped answering the phone, that fella had no one to say goodbye in hospital or his funeral. There were four people at the funeral, there should be 400.'

The pandemic also reinforced a broader problem, highlighted by the UK Commission on Bereavement (2022), that services often fail to reach groups and communities who may benefit from their support. The Commission emphasises in particular that: 'Those who identify as Black, Asian or another ethnic minority can struggle to find support that is culturally sensitive and tailored to their needs. Those who identify as non-binary, trans or are a member of the LBTQI+ community can also experience disenfranchised grief' (UK Commission on Bereavement, 2022). Our findings would suggest this experience has almost certainly increased over the course of the pandemic, with potentially long-term damage to the mental health of the bereaved as well as the communities of which they were part.

Looking to the future

In the autumn and winter of 2020–2021, organisations and community leaders working with older people had already demonstrated their ability to continue to meet the needs of their older members. However, the future for many organisations in the sector remained uncertain due to the continuation of social distancing (rules were eventually relaxed on 19 July 2021), and the emergence of new variants of COVID-19.

Organisations had lost funding, staff and volunteers, while demand for their services had increased at the same time. This new and evolving landscape was something to which they continued to respond while also trying to make plans for the future. Many referred to a 'culture shock' of having to adjust from years of an approach based on encouraging older people to come out of their homes to engage with others and their communities. After 12 months of social distancing, some older people were desperate to return to 'normal life' while others remained more cautious or even reluctant, as explained by

Figure 7.4: Hands together

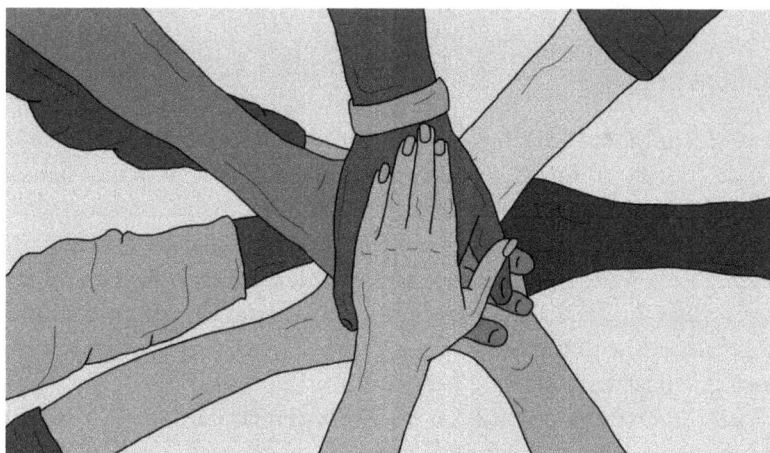

community organiser Joe: "Even if the government turns around and says we can forget about social distancing … can we forget about [face] masks? Can we forget about gloves? I think it's going to be about people's mindsets now in terms of how we go forward." This discussion has illustrated how many of the spaces of care within the community and voluntary sector were transferred to virtual ones. It remains to be seen how these will continue to be used, and their relationship with more traditional forms of social infrastructure within communities.

In 2021, many of the organisations in our research were starting to reintroduce face-to-face services. Often these were based on activities to help rebuild older people's confidence in order to re-engage in activities. Indoor activities proved to be difficult to reintroduce, as explained by community organiser Tracey: "The biggest challenge is going to be how we safely reopen the centre. We are going to have to grapple with risk assessments, guidelines, legal responsibilities and managing expectations from the public and staff, insurance and funding. On top of that there is the loss of income."

A key finding of this chapter was that although there were many strengths in the diversity of organisations we interviewed, inequalities existed in the level of resources which they were able to access. Although the age-friendly agenda was well co-ordinated by statutory services, those operating at the neighbourhood level were often limited in what they could do due to lack of funding and pre-existing inequalities. It is important to note that many local neighbourhoods included in this study had witnessed the hollowing-out of important social infrastructure, and were already experiencing precarity in terms of resources and facilities at the start of the pandemic. Concerns around funding and staff and volunteer shortages, and how older people would want to engage with services in the future, created an environment of considerable uncertainty for the majority of groups interviewed.

Conclusion

The community and voluntary sector formed an important landscape of care for older people in this study. The chapter has shown how the shape and form of this landscape was radically reorientated due to social distancing rules, which closed community spaces and vital social infrastructure. New virtual spaces of care were created to replace physical spaces such as community centres and libraries. Different services were developed to respond to changing needs within the population, especially where people experienced reduced contact with family and friends.

We also saw new relationships surface between virtual and physical spaces, and between formal and informal networks of support. Key individuals in neighbourhoods, who were often older people themselves, became central to maintaining support networks and complementing the work of formal organisations. As seen in Chapter 6, with regards to older people's personal relationships, the requirements of social distancing challenged how we understand the relationship between care and proximity. The people we interviewed at community and voluntary organisations cared deeply for their communities, often having built up long-standing relationships within them. From the onset of social distancing restrictions, and in many cases beforehand, they worked tirelessly to maintain a social, and often emotional, closeness with the older people they supported.

GM has a strong VCSE in general and has particular strengths in its network of age-friendly groups, organisations and services developed over several decades. Findings from this study show the creativity of the sector as well as the importance of being a part of the age-friendly networks in GM. Led by local government, the network supported collaboration and knowledge sharing to respond to the challenges in hand. The problems facing communities resulted in more informal networks emerging to support the activities of formal organisations. Although often associated in some way with formal organisations such as the GM Older People's Network or neighbourhood based community groups, people like Joyce or Martin also served as part of more informal contacts within their networks, often being the first point of contact for many other older people. These informal networks often proved vital in meeting the needs of the most marginalised and therefore support and recognition for such groups, and often individuals, will be crucial in a post-COVID-19 recovery.

Much has been made of the resilience of the community and voluntary sector in popular and academic discussions, together with its ability to demonstrate 'strength, creativity and innovation' during the pandemic

(British Academy, 2021: 10). While this chapter would certainly support findings around the creativity, ingenuity and pure stamina of the sector and individuals working within it, it would also argue that this only tells part of the story. By exploring the experience of organisations supporting older people in GM, more critical reflections on the experience of these organisations are also needed. The precarity of the sector must also be acknowledged, both through its changing role in relation to the state, the challenging economic conditions in which the sector has been operating, and the uncertainties faced by the communities it supports. Many of these organisations were financially vulnerable before the onset of COVID-19, an aspect that has intensified as a result of continued restrictions on public expenditure and the damage to social infrastructure inflicted by the pandemic.

8

Understanding everyday life during the pandemic

Introduction

Chapters 4 to 7 provided an overview of the range of experiences of everyday life under COVID-19 reported among our various groups of participants. This chapter reflects upon some of the *cross-cutting themes* which arose across the study, summarising the range of findings and observations which emerged from the interviews both with older people and community organisations. Chapter 9 builds on this overview and outlines a number of recommendations in relation to developing a 'community-centred approach' in responding to future variants of COVID-19, as well as making suggestions for how to create a post-pandemic neighbourhood.

A first observation is that, in many respects, older adults were no different from other age groups during the pandemic, managing as best they could, given the limits imposed on physical and social relationships. The interviews highlight the various ways in which older people tried to maintain their usual routines, in some cases, developing new interests and hobbies. Many participants were highly adaptable in their routines, whether through rediscovering interests in poetry, writing, arts and crafts, or befriending others via the medium of the telephone or online platforms. Some reflected on unexpected positive aspects of lockdown, such as being able to spend more time with their family, having the opportunity to focus on prayer or religious practice, or developing new digital skills. In this regard, our participants demonstrated a strong sense of agency, autonomy and creativity in managing what was an undoubted crisis affecting their daily lives (see also Fancourt et al, 2022).

The interviews with the community organisations also emphasised their inventiveness and adaptability. Existing services were frozen, and new types of support, such as telephone welfare checks and emergency food parcels offered, providing a much-needed emergency response to the pandemic. Over time, new services emerged, including online support groups, chair-based exercise sessions and well-being classes. Organisations also developed activities to cater for people unable to leave their homes and who had no means of engaging remotely. These included posting craft packs and telephone befriending. The age-friendly network developed in the region also provided a vital means of support and coordination for much of the work across GM.

However, at the same time, many organisations expressed concern that despite their best efforts at adapting services, not being able to host face-to-face activities undermined their ability to reach out to marginalised groups. While many offered emotional support, either online or via the telephone, the unprecedented circumstances of the pandemic and increased levels of need meant that some areas of concern were not being addressed. For organisations working with minority groups, such as those from the LGBTQ+ community, the inability to meet in physical spaces was particularly acute. Prior to the pandemic, LGBTQ+ friendly spaces were of particular importance in helping to reinforce a shared sense of identity and support within people's networks.

Role of technology

Adapting to, and exploiting *the benefits of technology*, was crucial for many of those interviewed. Indeed, an important finding from our work has been how the use of platforms such as Zoom entered into the language and rhythms of daily life. People spoke of digital technologies opening up opportunities to engage within their neighbourhoods; with family and friends in other countries (especially important for South Asian and African Caribbean communities); as a medium for sustaining their involvement in different social activities and religious practice; and as a source (particularly for the LGBTQ+ community) for reaffirming identity at a time when traditional forms of social contact were unavailable.

Those with resources and confidence in digital technology were able to transfer to online platforms to maintain activities and relationships with family and friends. Some participants 'regrouped' virtually to make up for what was no longer possible face-to-face, providing participants with vital companionship over the period of the three lockdowns. For some of those interviewed, the conditions of lockdown led to their first encounter with digital technology. Some learnt new skills, either through guidance provided by younger family members or neighbours (see Chapter 6) and/or support provided by community organisations (see Chapter 7). In these cases, digital technology often acted as an intergenerational medium that enhanced relationships and neighbourhood networks. Befriending services, whether online or by telephone, also offered a vital social link to many, particularly those living alone and those who were already at risk of social isolation.

Equally, it was clear that *those without access to online media* were disadvantaged in a variety of ways, notably in being unable to maintain contact with friends and family and in being deprived of services and activities that were only available online. Those lacking access to the internet experienced what Seifert et al (2021) refer to as a 'double burden of exclusion', with restrictions placed on physical contact compounded by inequalities in access to IT.

The community organisations interviewed became increasingly concerned that individuals and groups of older people who had been difficult to reach before the pandemic were now at an even greater risk of 'slipping through the net' due to digital exclusion and increased need. Differences in the use of technology through the pandemic has, we suggest, introduced *new forms of inequality within the older population*: an issue that would be a valuable subject for further research and policy consideration (see Chapter 9).

In our study, community organisations often played a crucial role in helping people living alone to get online during the pandemic, but the demand for their services was considerable. There was concern about services remaining online after the pandemic thereby exacerbating inequalities further. Before lockdown, these services provided vital support to those at risk of social isolation. The findings therefore demonstrate the need for a major public policy intervention to address digital exclusion, particularly in lower-income and minority communities, to help individuals to maintain social relationships in periods of crisis such as COVID-19 (Macdonald and Hülür, 2021).

Another observation from our research concerned the important *role of religion* in structuring and giving meaning to everyday life for some participants. Our interviewees came from a variety of faiths, including Methodist, Catholic, Quaker, Jehovah's Witness, Protestant, Evangelical, Pentecostal, Muslim, Sikh and Hindu. In many cases, faith and prayer were central to the organisation of daily life; in some cases, also providing a framework for making sense of the pandemic itself. Again, technology was an important medium in maintaining religious engagement, through the organisation of virtual church services and meetings of various kinds. Some interviewees mentioned how they had joined online worship across the world for the first time, thus extending their networks across international borders. Others described how members of their religious groups were like family, offering vital support and companionship throughout the 12-month period.

But it was also the case that many people spoke of missing social contacts and relationships gained through visiting their place of worship, with Zoom and related platforms often regarded as inadequate substitutes for face-to-face meetings. The impact of restricted numbers at funerals was also a major concern, and the inability to grieve and mourn properly resulted in considerable pain for many of those interviewed. Not being able to say goodbye to relatives during their final days, attend funeral services or visit the home of grieving friends and relatives was a major concern for many of the people we interviewed (see also UK Commission on Bereavement, 2022). Our findings show that it is likely that the impact of losing loved ones during the pandemic, and the sheer numbers of deaths affecting some communities, will be felt long into the future, with the psychological costs likely to have significant consequences for individual health and well-being as well as relationships within families and religious communities.

Issues and concerns relevant to the future care and support of older people

The interview findings illustrate the various means by which people managed their everyday lives during successive lockdowns, often finding innovative ways of maintaining links with their pre-pandemic lives. However, many participants reported existing health or social problems increased because of the various lockdowns. The next section reviews the most important of these, and the different types of changes encountered among the groups interviewed for our research. Here, we identify four main areas of concern: *ageing under lockdown*; *social isolation during the pandemic*; *relationships with family and friends*; and *the role of the home and neighbourhood during the crisis*, which form the basis for policy recommendations in Chapter 9.

Ageing under lockdown

An important finding from our research (highlighted in Chapter 4) concerned a degree of *physical and mental deterioration* affecting some of our participants over the duration of the research. Some spoke of the impact of restricted mobility over a number of months, because of being confined to their house or flat. The consequences included reduced confidence in getting around their neighbourhood or restarting exercise routines. For some of those interviewed, certain behaviours which were 'under control' before the pandemic became 'out of control' as COVID-19 progressed, for example, those relating to diet and alcohol consumption. In cases such as these, *the pandemic also seemed to increase awareness about ageing itself*, but often as a negative rather than positive life transition. Over the period of 12 months, many felt a loss of independence and were concerned about whether they would ever regain their confidence after lockdown restrictions were lifted. Some reported becoming more aware of the passing of time, and their own ageing, reinforced by having 'much less energy'; or feeling less physically or mentally able.

A related issue concerns the extent to which the pandemic may have *heightened* feelings of vulnerability among certain groups. An example from our research concerned those who had received a letter advising them to shield (see Chapter 4). Our findings show that in some cases, such guidance had a demoralising effect on mental health. It was indeed a shock for some to be told they were 'vulnerable'. This was not part of their self-image or how they defined themselves as a person. This may be another example where the pandemic will have a long-term (and potentially negative) impact on how many people think about their health and well-being coming out of lockdown. Perceptions of vulnerability may also be traced to other sources: people feeling they had become a 'burden' on their family or even on society itself. Among our South Asian and African Caribbean groups, racism may also have played a role; and within the LGBTQ+ group, discrimination and stigmatisation added to their sense of marginality or precariousness. Many of the community organisations also commented on what they viewed as the deterioration of older people's mental health and well-being among some groups during the pandemic, confirming findings from older people themselves.

Social isolation during the pandemic

Another observation from our research concerned the extent of *social isolation* arising from the pandemic, which was evident in some groups. There were particularly striking examples from some of the South Asian women interviewed for the study, and from White British men living alone (see Chapter 6). The issues were distinctive for each group but raise important questions for community support more broadly. Among the former, there were powerful expressions of the anguish caused by successive lockdowns, these resulting in feelings of depression, anxiety and being a 'prisoner in your own home'. Such sentiments were invariably driven by the increased pressures women felt as carers. Responsibilities – for example, caring for a sick husband – had remained the same, but support had weakened with social distancing and pressures on statutory services. We were struck by the intensity of the pressures experienced by these women – exacerbated in some cases by financial difficulties and poor housing. Single men living alone presented a contrasting set of issues, but with similar experiences of intense isolation among some of those interviewed. Prior to the pandemic, many of the single men had fragile social networks, poor physical health and low incomes. Those people who had experienced social exclusion and discrimination *before* the pandemic were often further disadvantaged as a result of COVID-19.

Successive lockdowns, in some cases, *disrupted routines created to ward off feelings of isolation*, or to fill the gap created by the loss of a partner. For others, being 'alone' over a sustained period created fresh anxieties: uncertainties about whether something was just an 'ordinary illness' or 'the virus'; worries about dying 'alone'; or having no one to put things in perspective: 'someone to talk to'. For some, spending 24 hours a day at home led them to reflect on the realities of living alone in a new light. 'Digital exclusion' was also a significant barrier to maintaining relationships, with the majority of those mentioning 'feeling worse' or more 'depressed' lacking access to different kinds of technology and social media.

Many of the interviewees mentioned key biographical *turning points* which influenced how they experienced or viewed the impact of COVID-19, such as the separation or death of a spouse, and for some of our gay participants, turning points related to reactions 'coming out' to their family and friends. As well as, in some cases, contributing to social isolation in later life, these turning points also provided some of the participants with resources to cope with the challenges brought about by COVID-19.

An additional pressure created by COVID-19 centred on the closure of vital social infrastructure, which many of the single men, in particular, invariably relied upon for support – community centres, local cafés, libraries and pubs. The loss of these facilities had a considerable impact and this emphasises their importance, especially within lower-income neighbourhoods.

Relationships with family and friends

What do we know, based on our interviews, about the impact of COVID-19 on *intimate ties*? To what extent did the pandemic *affect relationships with family and friends*? The study found that there were complex and uneven patterns of change that emerged from our interviews across the 12-month period, these being characterised as both *a contraction and expansion of social relationships* and *a reconfiguration of landscapes of care*.

In some cases, intimacy emerged in unexpected ways, as in the case of the befriending services that multiplied during the pandemic, or in different types of support provided by friends and neighbours who created 'support bubbles'. Our research also indicated the strains which could affect friendships as a result of social distancing. 'Not having much to talk about' was a typical comment and it illustrated a wider problem that the activities which sustain friendships – confiding, laughing together, sharing interests, providing emotional and instrumental support – could often only happen on a virtual basis. This worked in some cases for those who could adopt (or who had already adopted prior to the pandemic) technology as a way of maintaining relationships. Our findings confirmed how friends continued to play a crucial role throughout the 12-month period of the study. But for many, digitally included and excluded alike, keeping friendships going throughout the pandemic was a challenge.

There were examples of *relationships becoming more distant* and *some becoming closer*. Some participants developed new networks of support within changing landscapes of care. If friends became, in some cases, less proximate, *family was certainly centre-stage* for many of those we interviewed. Again, this was often the case among those most digitally connected, with Zoom and WhatsApp being drawn upon to maintain regular contact. Use of the internet to maintain *transnational ties* (almost certainly a feature of life before the pandemic) was an important element in the daily lives of many of our participants, particularly those from the African Caribbean and South Asian groups. However, for many, technology was a poor substitute for being physically present with family members, especially during difficult times.

For those women with significant caring responsibilities – our group of South Asian women were an obvious example – separation from family members outside the home was a major source of anxiety. Especially for those living in multigenerational households, there were tensions resulting from concerns about 'catching the virus' and passing it on to another member of the family. Our research also found that living with others did not always protect people from feeling isolated. Some relationships adapted while others flourished, but overall, intimate ties became more limited in a variety of ways.

For certain groups, the loss of friends may indeed be one long-term result of the pandemic. This may have a series of consequences for those affected, given evidence from research showing that friend relationships are as important as family ties in maintaining psychological well-being in adulthood and old age (Blieszner et al, 2019). In some cases, technology allowed people to expand their landscapes of care at a time when physical proximity was heavily restricted. Despite the fact relationships were enacted at a physical distance, there were examples of emotional closeness and social networks expanding. However, many worried about the long-lasting impact of the pandemic on their relationships and support networks.

The role of the home and neighbourhoods during the crisis

With people deprived of their usual routines and support networks, the home and social relationships in the immediate neighbourhood assumed greater importance during lockdown. Boundaries between the dwelling and neighbourhood were redefined, due to rules requiring people to stay 'at home'. Spaces outside and in between the home such as doorsteps, windows, garden fences and driveways became important places to drop off groceries and supplies, carry out welfare checks on those shielding, and for neighbours to catch up with each other. The neighbourhood also took on new significance, as a place of care and support for some, but with limited significance for others. Our interviews showed how for some participants, the opportunity to spend more time with family members or maintain usual routines was highly valued. In these accounts, the home was described as a sanctuary, a retreat away from the threats posed by the virus. In some cases, interviewees, particularly those who were shielding, became used to being at home and increasingly anxious about lockdowns ending. Some participants were fearful of having to mix in their neighbourhood again due to anxieties about the virus and concerns about the behaviour of others (see Chapter 4).

For some who were already at risk of isolation, the home was associated with negative emotions, a place where they felt increasingly bored, depressed and isolated over time. The restrictions made them feel like a 'prisoner' in their own home, for example, disturbed by noisy neighbours or increasingly concerned about the upkeep of their dwelling without vital support from family and friends (see Chapter 5). An important priority coming out of the pandemic will be addressing the need for decent and secure housing for those who have to shield again given the likely continuation of the virus in some form.

Among our participants, there were particular difficulties for some residents of sheltered housing schemes, who found themselves denied access to communal spaces such as gardens and laundry rooms – an experience viewed as 'infantilising' by many. The research highlighted how prior to the pandemic, many of the men relied on facilities in their local communities, what Oldenburg (1989) defines as 'third places', such as libraries, shopping centres and cafés, which encourage social interaction (Klinenberg, 2018). Lack of access to social infrastructure created considerable anxieties for many of those living alone, and the desire for the reopening of such facilities was a recurring theme. The pandemic itself, with the move to online shopping, combined with cuts in public expenditure which have led to the closure of libraries and community centres, may continue to create problems for those such as single older people who depend on such places to find company. Chapter 9 recommends that strengthening social infrastructure must be a priority, especially in those communities which have suffered the full force of the pandemic, combined with the effects of austerity and long-term multiple deprivation.

We noted the importance of access to *gardens, parks and communal spaces* in maintaining well-being for many of our participants. This was particularly significant from March through to early summer 2020, when spells of warm weather provided some relief from the pressures associated with the first lockdown. Connections to outdoor space were particularly important for managing extended periods of time alone. As confirmed in the research literature, those with access to a garden and/or a nearby park found these spaces especially beneficial (Lindley et al, 2020). Indeed, an important priority coming out of the pandemic will be addressing the negative impact of *unequal access to green space*.

While sources of community support were often celebrated during the pandemic, it is important to remember that this was not the experience of those living in transient or what were perceived as hostile neighbourhoods (see also Lewis and Buffel, 2020). The experience of these varied for different participants and between neighbourhoods. In some cases, experiences of racism or discrimination produced deeper feelings of alienation, with individuals less inclined to draw on the support of those living around them. In others, there was evidence for strong neighbourhood attachments predicated on informal social ties between neighbours which provided much needed support and access to resources for older people. For some participants who were isolated before the pandemic, being involved in a 'support bubble' cemented relationships with neighbours. It was notable that those neighbourhoods where such relationships existed were often well resourced in terms of community spaces and social infrastructure, around which networks of mutual aid could often be built.

The community organisations all commented on the loss of access to physical spaces when asked about the kind of facilities people were missing. Informal sites for socialising, often unstructured and without any expectation or obligation, have long played a vital role in supporting social networks for many community organisations. Fears were expressed that losing this type of social contact would further isolate individuals who were less confident about attending more formal groups.

Conclusion

Bringing together the findings from the study, this chapter has shown how the pandemic exposed the fragility of the pre-pandemic lives of some groups of older people, and the challenges faced in dealing with the crisis associated with COVID-19. The pandemic made people see existing spaces and engage with old activities in new ways, while simultaneously making underlying inequalities more apparent. It is certainly the case that for those detached from online communication, life was considerably restricted during the lockdowns. The possibility of these participants falling further behind as digital communication becomes a more important part of everyday life seems likely.

The findings also emphasise how many people were concerned about whether they would ever regain their independence after lockdown restrictions were lifted, particularly those who suffered from mental and physical health problems. Some reported how spending prolonged periods of time alone made them become more aware of the passing of time, and their own ageing. Unsurprisingly, many of our respondents experienced a steep decline in social contacts over the 12-month period and relationships with family and friends changed in numerous ways. In some cases, intimacy emerged in unexpected ways, and in other instances, relationships were lost, and networks of support became vanishingly small. The home and social relationships in the immediate neighbourhood assumed greater importance during lockdown, particularly access to gardens, parks and communal spaces for maintaining well-being and relationships. The neighbourhood also took on new significance, as places of care and support for some, but with limited significance for others. *Overall, the findings show how those who had experienced social isolation before the pandemic were often further disadvantaged as a result of COVID-19.* From this summary of the main findings from our research, we turn, in Chapter 9, to some recommendations in relation to policy and practice in the community, with some observations as well about potential areas for research.

9

COVID-19, inequality and older people: developing community-centred interventions

Introduction

In March 2020, our research began with tentative first steps in thinking about the likely impact that a new disease – SARS-CoV-2 (COVID-19) – might have on older populations, and in particular the communities in GM with whom we were already working. At the time of writing (December 2022), COVID-19 continues to have a serious impact on communities and health systems, coming in successive waves (rather than a seasonal cycle), and with the constant threat of new variants. Vaccinations have reduced the shockingly high death toll, but hundreds of people in the UK (mostly over 60) still die every week with COVID-19 mentioned as one of the causes, or are living with the consequences of the pandemic. In the week ending 9 December 2022 in England alone, 295 deaths were recorded involving COVID-19, 272 of whom were people aged 65 and over (ONS, 2022c) – the continued toll of deaths amongst older people still attracting relatively little official or media comment.

The aim of this book has been to document the way different groups of older people responded to the pandemic, with a particular focus on those living in urban neighbourhoods. Chapters 4 to 7 gave particular emphasis to understanding how people experienced COVID-19, in the context of their family and friends, homes, neighbourhoods, and wider social networks. These dimensions of everyday life are, invariably, the building blocks of people's lives. But at the same time, they are also the starting point for how we need to develop effective policies for supporting people during periods of crisis associated with pandemics such as COVID-19. In this chapter, we argue that preparation for pandemics in vital areas such as vaccine development and manufacture must also be complemented by direct engagement with the lived experiences of communities themselves – and especially those who are likely to be especially vulnerable to the effects of pandemics.

This chapter develops an argument for developing what we call 'community-centred' policies in the area of public health. The discussion is, first, situated in the context of debates around supporting 'ageing in place' and developing 'age-friendly cities and communities'. Second, we outline the basis for a 'community-centred' approach for tackling COVID-19. Third, we identify a series of recommendations for those engaged in developing urban health policies to tackle future waves of COVID-19 and similar pandemics.

Developing age-friendly communities

Policies in Europe have emphasised the role of the local environment in promoting 'ageing in place', a term used to describe the aim of helping people to remain in their own homes and neighbourhoods (rather than residential care) in later life (Wiles et al, 2012). The World Health Organization has been especially influential in raising awareness about how to adapt urban environments to the needs and preferences of people ageing in place, through the development of its 'Age-Friendly Cities and Communities' project. Alley et al define an age-friendly city as a 'place where older people are actively involved, valued, and supported with infrastructure and services that effectively accommodate their needs' (2007: 4). In 2010, the World Health Organization launched the Global Network of Age-Friendly Cities and Communities, which by 2023 had reached a membership of around 1,400 cities and communities in 44 countries across the Global North and South.

The period from the mid-2000s saw a substantial growth of interest in age-friendly issues, with a variety of projects and achievements linking ageing populations to the need for changes to the built and social environment, transportation, housing and neighbourhood design (World Health Organization, 2018; Stafford, 2019; van Hoof et al, 2021). However, a combination of widening inequalities within and between urban environments, and the impact of austerity on local government and city budgets, has raised questions about future progress in developing age-friendly programmes and related activities (Buffel et al, 2018).

To these pressures, the impact of COVID-19 should now be added, with the pandemic having its greatest impact (as highlighted in Chapter 2) on areas characterised by high levels of deprivation, often with ageing populations, poor quality housing and communities experiencing long-term decline through deindustrialisation (Beatty and Fothergill, 2021). Buffel et al (2021) suggest that under social distancing guidelines, older people living in socio-economically deprived urban neighbourhoods experienced a 'double lockdown' as a result of interrelated social and spatial inequalities associated with COVID-19. Yet, despite the known pressures on low-income communities, little was done to inject extra resources into these communities at the start of the pandemic, or to engage directly with organisations working with some of the most vulnerable and excluded groups in such areas (Marmot et al, 2020; Munford et al, 2022).

Both elements need urgent consideration if there is to be greater protection from the impact either of the continuation of COVID-19 or from future pandemics. In what follows, emphasis is given to the importance of close engagement with communities, viewed in the context of a redistribution of financial resources in favour of lower-income areas. This should be seen as a pre-condition for developing effective policies for tackling the social and geographical inequalities associated with the impact of COVID-19.

Community participation and COVID-19

The argument of this chapter is that communities have, to date, been marginalised in strategies to combat COVID-19. Christakis (2020) highlights two broad ways to respond to pandemics: first, pharmaceutical interventions (PIs), such as medications and vaccinations; second, non-pharmaceutical interventions (NPIs) which are either individual (for example, mask-wearing, self-isolating) or collective (for example, shutting schools, banning large gatherings). To date, collective NPIs have largely comprised of actions led by government, delivering messages, for example, through press conferences, the internet, social media platforms and the national press. These interventions have been complemented by the work of regional and local authorities, in many cases using networks developed prior to the pandemic. However, the evidence suggests that neighbourhoods and the different groups within them have been at the receiving end of actions to combat COVID-19, rather than being treated as equal partners. As Marston et al note: '[these actions] have largely involved government telling communities what to do, seemingly with minimal community input' (2020: 1676).

Absent in current NPIs is the type of community-centred model put forward by Public Health England, which suggests that:

> Community (or citizen) participation, that is the active involvement of people in formal or informal activities, programmes and/or discussions to bring about planned change or improvements in community life, services and/or resources, has long been a central tenet of public health and health promotion. ... There is a compelling case for a shift to more people and community-centred approaches to health and well-being. The core concepts that underpin this shift are voice and control, leading to people having a greater say in their lives and health; equity, leading to a reduction in avoidable inequalities, and social connectedness, leading to healthier more cohesive communities. (Public Health England, 2015: 8–9)

Yet, these principles were not implemented in the development of COVID-related NPIs, notably in the type of approach from central government, with PIs, and vaccines in particular, presented as the 'magic bullet' for managing the pandemic, as opposed to being integrated with neighbourhood-focused activities. A number of reasons can be identified for bringing communities to the forefront of future strategies. Marston et al make the general point that:

> [C]ommunities, including vulnerable and marginalised groups can identify solutions: they know what knowledge and rumours are circulating; they can provide insights into stigma and structural barriers; and they are well-placed to work with others from their communities to devise collective solutions. Such community participation matters because unpopular measures risk low compliance. With communities on side, we are more likely—together—to come up with innovative, tailored solutions that meet the full range of needs of our diverse populations. (Marston et al, 2020: 1676)

Targeting low-income areas with tailored public health messages is essential because of the 'clustering' of 'at risk' groups. The evidence suggests that areas with a concentration of overcrowded housing had the worst outcomes from COVID-19. The Centre for Ageing Better (2020) in association with The King's Fund, reporting on the first wave of the pandemic, found that of the 20 local authorities with the highest COVID-19 mortality rate, 14 had the highest percentage of households living in homes with fewer bedrooms than needed.

One of the weaknesses in current approaches of working with older people is an over-reliance on access to the internet as a means of communication. This ignores the extent of digital exclusion among particular groups – notably, but not exclusively, the older population. In 2020, according to ONS (2020) figures, 11.4 per cent of people aged 65–74 had never used the internet, with this figure rising to 38.8 per cent for those aged 75 and over. These age groups are likely to be further disadvantaged by the decline of local newspapers – 265 closed in the UK in the period 2005–2020 (Tobitt, 2020). Given this context, more traditional means of communication about COVID-19 and future pandemics will most probably be necessary (for example, leaflets in different languages through doors; advertising in shops) to complement digital communication and related approaches.

In addition, developing a community-centred approach is important in *convincing people that their own actions really can make a difference.* Christakis makes the point that:

> If we see pandemics purely as a function of biological details ... we may be lulled into thinking there is nothing we can do to prevent or arrest such events. But if we see pandemics as sociological phenomena as well, we can more clearly recognize the role of human agency. And the more we see our own role in shaping the emergence and unfolding

of pandemic diseases, the more proactive and effective our responses can be. (Christakis, 2020: 316)

The next section of this chapter considers how a community-centred strategy might be developed, one which acknowledges the long-term impact that the pandemic is likely to have, especially for those vulnerable due to their age, ethnicity or living in an area of high deprivation.

Community-centred strategies and tackling COVID-19

This section addresses the question of how to develop specific strategies which can strengthen the impact of NPIs but also facilitate (where necessary) the uptake of PIs. These proposals should be viewed as a contribution to developing a new public health strategy focused on protecting lower-income communities. The focus of the discussion will be on older adults, but the examples given are relevant to other age groups as well. The areas covered include: *promoting community participation*; *recruiting advocates for those who are isolated and/or socially excluded*; *developing social infrastructure*; *creating a national initiative for supporting community-centred activity*; and *developing long-term community-centred policies*.

Promoting community participation

What might community empowerment mean given the importance of protecting people against either future variants of COVID-19 or its equivalent? Our approach to participation is that it is more than just about 'consulting', 'involving' or 'engaging' people. Instead, the emphasis should be on renegotiating power and building capacities to help people gain more control over the neighbourhoods in which they live. Some potential areas of work here include: first, drawing on collaborative methods of co-research, as developed, for example, by Blair and Minkler (2009), Buffel (2019) and others. Older people, trained in research skills, are best placed to play a vital role in: deepening our understanding of attitudes towards COVID-19 – especially among groups experiencing various forms of social exclusion; assisting dissemination of advice and messaging about protection from the virus; and challenging negative stereotypes of older people by emphasising the skills and knowledge which they can bring to support work to control the virus.

Second, working with 'informal' and 'formal' leaders within communities could assist the uptake of PIs and encourage people to stay as safe as possible. The importance of this has increased given evidence about misleading/ false information spread through social media, notably about the benefits of vaccines. One example of the central role of community leaders was evident

Figure 9.1: Intergenerational exchange

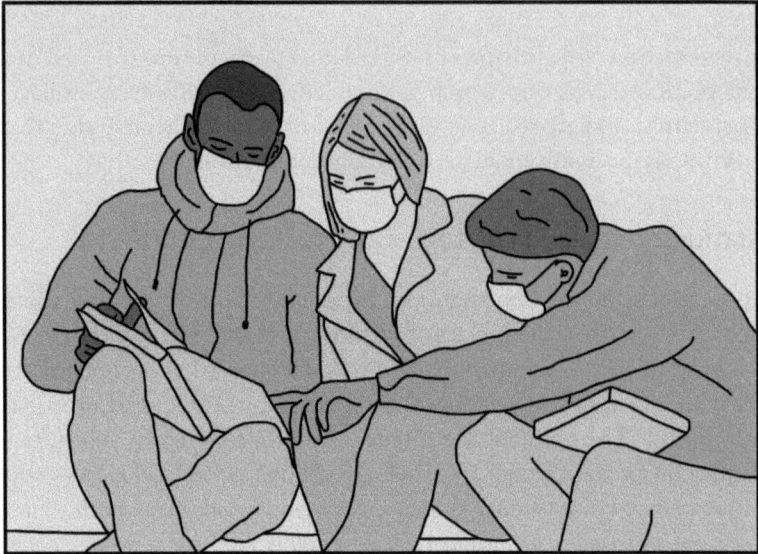

in January 2021 when a group of imams delivered sermons in mosques across the UK which sought to reassure worshippers about the safety and legitimacy of COVID-19 vaccinations and remind them of the Islamic injunction to save lives (Sherwood, 2021). The move came amid evidence of anxiety within Muslim communities about the roll-out of vaccines, and concern about slow take-up in some parts of the UK. The Scientific Advisory Group for Emergencies concluded that:

> Community engagement can identify strategies to make the vaccine more accessible, including in settings outside of formal health service provision, and increases trust between formal organisations and community members. This requires involving community leaders as partners ... to promote local buy-in and develop community plans. ... Community forums that address the cultural and historical context of vaccine research mistreatment and including diverse representation of stakeholders can increase trust. (Scientific Advisory Group for Emergencies, 2020: 7)

Third, building on existing networks and neighbourhood organisations will be vital in developing community-based interventions. Again, this can be through both 'informal' and 'formal' networks. Gardner (2011) highlights the importance of what she terms 'natural neighbourhood networks'. These refer to the 'web of informal relationships and interactions that enhance well-being and shape the everyday social world of older people ageing in place' (Gardner, 2011: 263). Gardner's research demonstrates the importance of 'third spaces' for older people (for example, informal sites such as cafés, local businesses, libraries and local streets), all of which must be considered essential facilities for conveying information and supporting people during the pandemic.

In terms of formal networks, the UK Network of Age-Friendly Communities, supported by the Centre for Ageing Better, has 55 members across the four UK countries. Many of these networks implemented important initiatives to support people during the pandemic, including campaigns to challenge ageist narratives, developing innovative forms of social participation, and distributing information booklets targeted at older people who are not online (Centre for Ageing Better, 2020). This work was supported in a number of areas in England by the local partnerships formed through the National Lottery-funded 'Ageing Better' programme, which ran from 2015 to 2022. 'Ageing Better' was designed to tackle problems relating to loneliness and social isolation among older people, with a particular focus on people living in low-income neighbourhoods (McKenna et al, 2022). The variety of projects and initiatives developed by the programme, with their emphasis on co-production and improving social connections, provides an important resource for developing community-based approaches to public health (Yarker and Buffel, 2022).

Recruiting community advocates

The second area for intervention concerns recruiting 'community advocates' for those who may not have anyone who can speak on their behalf. In reality, many older adults are able to safeguard their interests or have a 'convoy of support' (family, friends, neighbours) who are able to intercede on their behalf. However, there are increasing numbers in the population who may be having their interests ignored at times of crisis such as COVID-19. Klinenberg, in research on the impact of the 1995 Chicago heat wave, pointed to the rise of an ageing population of urban residents living alone: 'often without proximate or reliable sources of routine contact and social support' (Klinenberg, 2002: 230). He pointed, in particular, to problems faced by older men who had outlived 'their social networks or become housebound and ill, often suffer[ing] from social deprivation and role displacement in their later years' (Klinenberg, 2002: 230; see Chapter 6, this volume).

The issue identified by Klinenberg has undoubtedly become more serious in the intervening years – with a growth in the population of men and women living alone, in circumstances where accessing help has become increasingly difficult. Beach and Bamford (2014), using data from the English Longitudinal Study of Ageing, found that 14 per cent of older men experienced moderate to high social isolation compared to 11 per cent of women. Almost one in four older men (23 per cent) had less than monthly contact with their children,

Figure 9.2: Sharing food

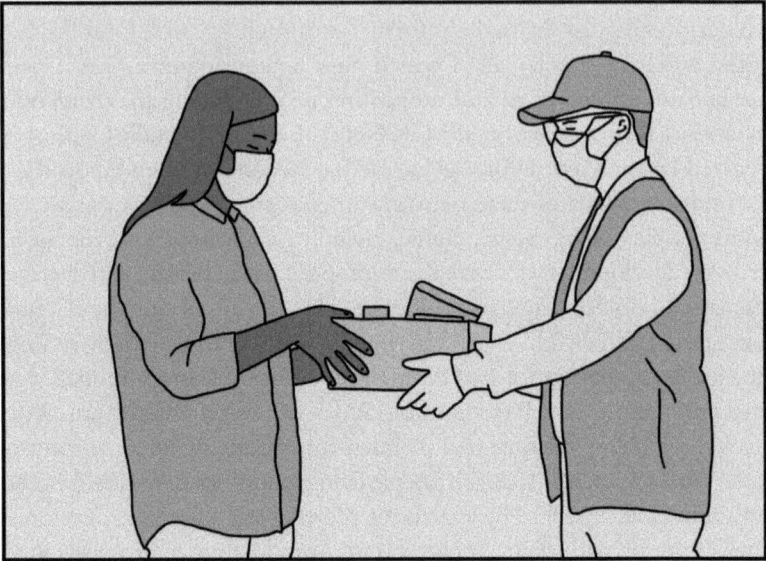

and close to one in three (31 per cent) had less than monthly contact with other family members. For women, these figures were 15 per cent and 21 per cent, respectively. The authors concluded that as the population of older men continues to grow and more people in this group find themselves living alone, social isolation and the potential issues it brings are set to get worse.

Social isolation need not necessarily be such an acute problem if services are plentiful and easily available. However, the combination of austerity and COVID-19 has drastically rationed support of all kinds – the impact of which may be especially severe for isolated men who may, in any event, according to Beach and Bamford (2014), be less likely to seek medical or other forms of help when needed. In this situation, and given the long-term pressures which health and social care are likely to experience, developing a network of advocates within communities will be important to prevent isolated individuals being denied appropriate treatment and support. Advocates could be drawn from existing organisations, for example local Age UK branches, Good Neighbours and befriending groups. However, this would require resourcing for training and financial support to those carrying out such work, an issue considered in further detail in the following section.

Developing social infrastructure

A key recommendation from this study is that investing in community-based services and organisations will be vital in ensuring social, psychological and practical support for marginalised and vulnerable groups. Government allocations of funding to the voluntary and community sector will need to increase, and the resilience of neighbourhoods, already weakened before the pandemic, will require strengthening (Marmot et al, 2020). Alongside community-based capacity building and supporting local initiatives, investing in the physical and institutional infrastructure of cities is crucial. The development and maintenance of social connections should also form a key part of recovery strategies to build back fairer communities (Marmot et al, 2020; Manchester City Council, 2022). The social support generated in spaces such as libraries and community centres has been found to be protective of health and well-being across the life course (Cotterell et al, 2018; Hertz, 2020).

Building on Klinenberg's (2018) research on the importance of social infrastructure, Finlay and her colleagues make the point that such community spaces 'represent essential sites to address society's pressing challenges, including isolation, crime, education, addiction, physical inactivity, malnutrition, and socio-political polarization' (Finlay et al, 2019: 2). Social infrastructure is essential in the recovery from the COVID-19 pandemic for promoting social connections, community cohesion, and for continuing to support age-friendly communities. Installing designated age-friendly benches in parks, ensuring seating to allow people to queue comfortably in shops and promoting accessible, green, safe and inviting public spaces, are just a few examples of how 'age-friendly' interventions may address the needs of different age groups (Yarker, 2022a).

National funding

The fourth argument is for a national, government-funded initiative to support community-centred work. Marston et al make the case for funding community engagement taskforces to ensure that a community voice is incorporated into responses to pandemics such as COVID-19. They argue that this will require:

> [D]edicated staff who can help governments engage in dialogue with citizens, work to integrate the response across health and social care, and coordinate links with other sectors such as policing and education. This engagement will require additional resources to complement existing health services and public health policy. Dedicated virtual and physical spaces must be established to co-create the COVID-19 response, with different spaces tailored to the needs of different participants—e.g., different formats for discussion, timings, locations, and levels of formality. (Marston et al, 2020: 1677)

Some areas may already have taskforces working along these lines, but the need both for additional funding from central government, and the importance of raising the profile of community-centred work, will be vital. This work will be especially important in developing effective policies over the longer term, given the possibility of a return of high levels of COVID-19 and the re-adoption of social distancing in some form. The implications of this last point are addressed in more detail in the final section of this chapter.

Developing long-term community-centred policies

Finally, the impact of COVID-19 can be measured in a variety of ways – in terms of reduced quality of life, lost income, mortality and long-term illness. Reflecting on all these, we know that the pandemic has already accelerated the decline in life expectancy which had started to affect poorer areas in England and Wales over the period 2010–2020 (Aburto et al, 2021). We also know, as outlined at the beginning of this chapter, that COVID-19 remains an ever-present danger in the community, especially for people aged 65 and over, who remain the majority of those dying from COVID-19 or subject to long-term serious illness. Accepting COVID-19 as an ever-present part of the community is consistent with views about the interaction between diseases and long-term patterns of global social and community change.

Christakis (2020) makes the point that COVID-19 needs to be placed within the wider context of globalisation, mass migrations and increased urbanisation with these factors contributing to the persistence of infectious diseases. He argues that:

> Outbreaks of novel pathogens reflect, among other things, changes in the way in the way humans come into contact with animals. In fact, two of the biggest challenges humans face—extreme weather events ... and periodic outbreaks of serious diseases—may be linked by climate change. People driven from their homes by changes in the weather or people clearing new land for cultivation may come into contact with animals (who may also be driven from their homes) in ways that increase the likelihood of the emergence of new pathogens in our species. (Christakis, 2020: 298–299)

However, it should also be noted that increased instability in the world coincides with the rise in populations (such as those comprising people over 60) who are especially vulnerable to infectious diseases. COVID-19 (or some variant) is likely to persist for some time for a variety of reasons (Horton, 2021). PIs – for those countries that can afford them – will certainly be vital in controlling the spread of the virus. At the same time, as commentators such as Christakis (2020) have pointed out, many 'unknowns' remain: their affordability (for many countries); their efficacy against new mutations; and their supply. Given this context, developing neighbourhood-level public health systems will be essential to run alongside successive programmes of vaccinations. Developing this argument, three priorities might be highlighted.

First, community-centred work needs to be understood within a wider context of 'community development'. COVID-19 has preyed on neighbourhoods damaged by cuts to basic services and social infrastructure, lack of investment in housing, and the rise of precarious forms of employment. Any long-term strategy to combat the pandemic must address the multiple forms of deprivation affecting many communities in the UK. These, as the evidence shows, are drivers for transmission of the virus, notably through overcrowded households, with members employed in high-risk occupations passing the virus across generations (Scientific Advisory Group for Emergencies, 2020).

However, community development must also come from 'below', with the pandemic giving impetus to what Sennett refers to as 'localised sociability', assisted by the strengthening of neighbourhood-based organisations (Sennett, 2020: 143). This may be especially important given the impact of successive lockdowns in potentially reinforcing social isolation among some groups. The effects of successive lockdowns remain unclear: for example, in creating a loss of confidence in moving around neighbourhoods; re-establishing relationships; and developing new contacts. One possible consequence will be the need to establish new forms of solidarity within communities, drawing on the collective organisation of older people. Relevant examples which emerged before the pandemic include the 'Village' movement, and Naturally Occurring Retirement Communities (both developed in the United States), and consolidation of the World Health Organization's global network of age-friendly cities and communities (Buffel et al, 2018). These, and other approaches, provide useful models for the direct involvement of older people in rebuilding communities in which they are likely to have spent a significant part of their adult life.

Second, COVID-19, as numerous reports have made clear, has exposed and exacerbated long-standing inequalities affecting BAME groups in the UK. Racism and discrimination also played an important role in this regard, as highlighted in research cited in Chapter 2. However, the impact of institutional racism and inequality in exposing ethnic minority people to higher rates of COVID-19 was predictable, given available knowledge about poverty, co-morbidities, poor-quality housing and low incomes affecting many of those in South Asian and other BAME communities. The question is why there was a failure to develop preventative forms of community-centred working with BAME groups from the start of the pandemic. Such targeted work, involving community leaders wherever possible, will certainly be essential over the medium and longer term. However, as suggested earlier, this type of initiative will require additional sources of funding to support what are financially constrained organisations even in 'normal times'.

Third, as observed in Chapter 2, COVID-19 has proved catastrophic for people in residential care – in the UK as well as for many other countries. By mid-January 2021 in the UK, one-third of fatalities were among care home residents – 32,000 people after taking into account those who had died after being admitted to hospital (Booth and McIntyre, 2021). This is an extraordinary figure, which indicates a *systemic* failure to safeguard a highly vulnerable group. Bold thinking is certainly needed by the research and policy community about the future of residential and nursing home care: challenging rather than colluding with current models of care. Privatisation has proved a flawed model; but the public or not-for-profit sector does not provide a straightforward solution either. The way forward must certainly be to 'downsize' from 'industrial-scale' care, potentially looking at placing the management of homes within a local authority framework. Crucially, such homes should be embedded in their surrounding neighbourhood. Developing viable models which provide some degree of protection for people will be challenging, but the impact of COVID-19 has confirmed the urgent need for major reforms of the residential and nursing home sector.

Conclusion

COVID-19 has presented a defining public health challenge for the 21st century. The issues identified in this chapter underline the need to implement a community-based strategy which foregrounds values of empowerment, anti-ageism and anti-racism. The devastating impacts of COVID-19 must prompt us to rethink the kind of infrastructure needed to support vulnerable populations in times of crisis. For older people – as with other groups – the consequences of the pandemic have weakened the 'informal' networks which sustain everyday life. But the effects have been amplified for those living in socio-economically deprived neighbourhoods where austerity and now COVID-19 have had the greatest impact.

The task now is to find solutions to the issues posed by the pandemic, and to ensure that older people are active participants in developing the new public health policies necessary for the years ahead. Communities demonstrated considerable resilience through the various periods of lockdown associated with COVID-19. But the combination of austerity and cuts to welfare programmes, along with the damage inflicted by the pandemic, has meant considerable work will be required to restore the physical and social infrastructure of communities. This chapter has set out some of the key steps for involving communities themselves in this process, an essential next step in the process of 'building back fairer' from COVID-19 and its aftermath.

10

Conclusion

The aim of this book has been to further understanding of the impact of COVID-19 on the *everyday life and relationships of older people*, together with the organisations working on their behalf. As outlined in Chapter 2, one result of the pandemic has been to greatly strengthen approaches which view ageing from a biomedical perspective. As a consequence, the broader cultural, economic and social forces which influence later life have yet to be given sufficient attention in discussions about the impact of the pandemic. This concluding chapter draws together the main arguments presented in the book, highlighting the challenges and responses of older people over three successive lockdowns starting in March 2020.

The discussion is organised as follows: first, the chapter summarises the *sociological approach* developed to understand the implications of the pandemic for older people; second, the *interdisciplinary framework* used to analyse the findings in each chapter is presented; third, some of the opportunities and challenges of the *methodological design* of the study are discussed; fourth, some *future areas of research* are outlined; and, finally, the arguments presented in the book are linked to broader issues arising from living in a more *precarious world*, one associated with the impact of developments such as climate change as well as the possibility of future pandemics.

Lived experience of the pandemic

The research set out to explore the '*lived experience*' of older people, drawn from a variety of neighbourhoods across GM, and from different social and ethnic groups aged 50 and upwards. The study also examined responses from a variety of voluntary and community organisations, highlighting the impact of social distancing and lockdowns on the management of services. The interviews provided detailed accounts of the ways in which older people and community groups experienced the impact of COVID-19 *over different points in time*, in the context of their family and friends, homes, neighbourhoods and wider social networks. The book argues that insights from these observations must form the starting point for how we understand the changing needs of older groups in their communities, as well as develop effective policies for supporting people during a period of crisis such as that represented by COVID-19 (see Chapter 9).

Everyday life is what we assume to be mundane, familiar and unremarkable, but as our findings show, the everyday matters because it offers 'angles and lenses' to explore tensions between the seen and unseen as well as between macro structures and local interactions (Yates, 2022). Our research, for example, provides new insights into the ways in which intimate ties within the household were reoriented during the pandemic, and how some caring relationships were placed under considerable strain, in the context of pressures from reduced health and social care support. Our focus on the everyday also demonstrates the agency of individuals in their daily lives, as well as forms of resistance, with a particular emphasis on 'feelings and experience' (Highmore, 2002: 5). In many cases, our participants demonstrated a strong sense of autonomy and creativity in managing a period of crisis both for themselves and the social networks of which they were a part.

The analysis in this book also focused on the importance of relationships in daily life, showing how the ways in which people make sense of the world, and live their everyday lives, are fundamentally shaped by *connections to other people* (May and Nordqvist, 2019). Our research explored the various ways in which these connections changed over the course of the lockdowns, bringing greater intensity to some relationships while withdrawal from others. The study also showed the creative way in which people made great efforts to maintain social ties, for example through the use of technology and online platforms of various kinds.

As well as providing a detailed account of the ways that people organised their everyday lives and supported others in their households and neighbourhoods, the book also showed how the pandemic placed a 'spotlight' on the precarity and unmet needs of some groups of older adults, such as those living alone, or from ethnic minority backgrounds. Overall, our findings support Portacolone et al's (2021) argument that COVID-19 *amplified* existing insecurities, as the pandemic exposed the fragility of pre-pandemic lives of some older people and the challenges they faced in dealing with the crisis associated with the pandemic. Extending this argument further, it might be argued that the pandemic *introduced new vulnerabilities*, exacerbating further the precarious lives of some groups of older people.

Overall, the book outlines a *sociological approach* for understanding the implications of the pandemic, revealing how existing inequalities between social and ethnic groups interacted with COVID-19, in many cases, with long-lasting effects. Each chapter focused on different dimensions of daily life during lockdown, and drew on an *interdisciplinary* approach to analyse the findings. Chapter 2 proposed a theoretical framework for understanding the pressures facing older people in the context of a more 'precarious' society. The discussion emphasised the importance of considering the *social context* affecting ageing populations, together with the impact of the pandemic on different groups of older people. Chapter 3 presented the *methodology* used in the study, explaining the qualitative longitudinal approach; how the sample was selected and recruited as well as the data analysis, using longitudinal and cross-sector approaches. Some context about the case study for the research, GM, was also provided.

Chapter 4 explored the impact of the pandemic and subsequent lockdowns on *everyday life*, over time. The discussion focused on themes including: the impact of shielding; social distancing and social isolation; growing old under lockdown; and reflections on the impact of COVID-19. Overall, the findings showed how people 'made do' in various ways in coping with the pandemic: through existing hobbies or new interests; spending more time on prayer and reflection; housework and gardening. Chapter 5 emphasised how our participants' *biographies* and *everyday life prior to COVID-19* influenced how they made sense of the pandemic. The four case studies reveal how the participants entered the pandemic through contrasting pathways, drawing on a range of resources and strategies to cope with what proved for many a transformative period of their lives. The analysis emphasised the importance of key biographical *turning points* which influenced how the impact of COVID-19 was viewed and experienced. Chapter 6 showed how *relationships and caring responsibilities* were reorientated due to social distancing rules, using a theoretical framework of landscapes of care. The analysis considered the different spaces through which caring relationships were experienced, as well as the different spatial patterns that emerged due to social distancing.

Chapter 7 examined the role of *community organisations* in GM which provided support to different groups of older people. The analysis considered the critical role of social infrastructure in providing support to older people, and the consequences arising from cuts to facilities over the last decade. The findings were analysed in relation to broader discussion about the precarity faced by both older people and the organisations that support and work with them. Chapter 8 highlighted how these multidimensional accounts of everyday life support a better understanding of the full impact of COVID-19 on older people, the organisations working on their behalf, and the communities in which they live. Two main elements of the findings were highlighted: *general experiences of daily life under the pandemic* and *issues and concerns relevant to the future care and support of older people*. Chapter 9 presented the case for developing a *community-centred approach* in responding to COVID-19 and future variants. A number of recommendations were outlined, in relation to developing a 'community-centred approach' in responding to future variants of COVID-19, as well as making suggestions for how to create post-pandemic neighbourhoods.

Reflections on the design of the study

In order to uncover the breadth and diversity of experiences and subjective responses to the pandemic, the study used a *qualitative longitudinal approach* (see also Settersten et al, 2020). As Vindrola-Pandros and colleagues suggest, in the context of the pandemic, such research can uncover experiences which complement epidemiological data 'by providing insights into people's lived experience of disease, care, and epidemic response efforts' (Vindrola-Pandros et al, 2020: 2194). One of the advantages of the *longitudinal approach* was being able to identify changes affecting *people over time*. In our case, a period which captured three successive lockdowns from March 2020 to early 2021. This longitudinal approach opened-up opportunities for generating a critical understanding of change over time (May, 2018), such as how the community and voluntary sectors' responses evolved over the 12-month period.

Studying the *experiences* of people during a pandemic is novel, as most research tends to be carried out after the event which is the focus of concern (Portacolone et al, 2021). Interviewing during COVID-19 produced both opportunities and limitations. *Telephone interviews* enabled us to provide time-sensitive accounts of individual experiences of the pandemic, when understanding rapid social change was of vital importance (Tarrant et al, 2021). Because the interviews were carried out on the telephone from home, some participants reflected that they felt at ease and comfortable being in a familiar environment, and enjoyed the opportunity to reflect on the pandemic, when social contact was heavily restricted. However, the research team were concerned about the potential negative impact of speaking about stressful events, and were also unable to capture the unspoken elements of conversations, such as hand gestures and body language which are an important dimension of face-to-face interviews. Overall, the use of telephone interviews was highly effective for working during the pandemic restrictions and engaging with hard to reach groups. However, in future research, we would emphasise the importance of using *collaborative or co-research approaches* to ensure that older people have a closer involvement with the research process (Buffel, 2019).

Throughout the duration of the study, the project team held regularly discussions with a *Research Advisory Board* consisting of people who worked with older people from a range of neighbourhoods and backgrounds. The Board provided helpful guidance on each part of the research process, including the recruitment of participants, the format for the interviews and the dissemination of findings. By collaborating with organisations who work with minority groups, the research team were able to recruit participants from a variety of backgrounds and to tailor the research questions so they were culturally sensitive. Some of the interviews with the South Asian participants were carried out by the partner organisations in other languages, thereby including older people who are often not included in research.

The project team are indebted to a network of *community organisations* who assisted with the research. We were able to respond swiftly to news of the emerging crisis in spring 2020 and benefited greatly from working with community and voluntary organisations and their existing networks across

GM, including those working in particular neighbourhoods, or specific minority communities of identity or experiences. With guidance from these organisations, we were able to promptly plan a programme of community-based research to assess the early responses to the pandemic, and how they changed over the 12-month period. The team are also grateful for the input of statutory services and local authorities across the region. In particular, Greater Manchester Combined Authority Ageing Hub provided funding and extensive help and support throughout the project. And lastly, we would like to thank the Manchester Urban Ageing Research Group (MUARG) for their input and support with the wider study.

The *sample* (102 people, aged 50 and over) were not chosen 'randomly', rather, they were identified by community organisations on the basis of particular characteristics that left them at risk of social isolation such as living in a lower-income neighbourhood and being a member of a particular social or ethnic group. As a result, our study was intentionally not about the *general experiences* of older people across GM. Instead, we view our work as *complementing* local, regional and national surveys, by looking in greater depth at how *particular* groups of people maintained a sense of *agency* and well-being. Also, how they made sense of and interpreted the pandemic; the differing *resources and capacities* they had available to help alleviate the pressures of the pandemic; and how this *varied* according to categories such as household composition, ethnicity, sexuality, gender and age cohort. Our findings drew attention to some of the particular issues relevant to different groups. There were, of course, limitations to our sample. Since recruitment was carried out in collaboration with community organisations, we were not able to include those who were severely socially isolated and not in contact with any services. Also, interviews were conducted by telephone, thereby excluding those with hearing impairments or other disabilities which might restrict use of the telephone. An important area of future research would be to understand the impact of the pandemic on these groups.

Future areas of research

There are a number of issues arising from our study which indicate some priority areas for future research. We would emphasise four in particular: first, *understanding changes affecting communities*; second, *developing work on the experiences of older people from ethnic minority groups*; third, *researching the impact of digital inequalities*; and, fourth, *challenging ageism*.

On the first of these, an important question for research is: *how can we strengthen relationships and infrastructure within communities, ahead of any future pandemics?* The British Academy (2021) highlighted three important developments which were affecting communities before the pandemic: a slow decline in people's sense of neighbourhood belonging; a shift to people finding a sense of community in virtual spaces and online; and loss of funding for social infrastructure in the form of libraries, community centres and post offices. An important question for research is: *how far were these trends consolidated, accelerated or even reversed as a result of the pandemic?*

One positive result of the pandemic, highlighted by our findings, was the emergence in many instances of new relationships within communities, with the development of 'support bubbles', mutual aid groups, informal networking in neighbourhoods, and the spread of different kinds of online forums. But we know very little about whether these developments are likely to be *sustained* over the longer term, or whether they were stronger in some communities compared with others. Another set of questions concerns whether communities were *selective* in their responses to the pandemic, operating on the basis of pre-established networks and resources, thus potentially excluding marginalised groups, the socially isolated or those resistant to seeking help (Lorenz and Dittmer, 2022). These issues should be considered in a programme of research which compares pandemic responses in different types of communities, with contrasting demographic and social characteristics.

A second major issue for research concerns responding to the experiences of ethnic minority communities during the various waves of the pandemic. Chapter 2 examined the range of inequalities experienced by different groups, reflecting the interaction of racism with pre-existing social and economic conditions relating to poverty, inadequate housing and insecure employment. Ethnic minority groups were acutely vulnerable to the effects of COVID-19, whether through higher rates of mortality affecting their community, long-term illness, the effects of overcrowded housing or the nature of their employment. Yet none of the factors which increased the exposure of different groups have gone away. Indeed, given factors such as the long-term decline in wages, the pressures on health and social care, the cost of living crisis, and inadequate housing in inner-city areas, such groups may be even more 'at risk' in the future.

This suggests an urgent need for research which can examine questions such as: *how can ethnic minority groups be better protected from variants of COVID-19 and impending pandemics? What are the variations between and within different groups in terms of their vulnerability? How can the racism which affects access to health care and related services be best tackled?* Such questions will need to be considered through an interdisciplinary programme of research, but one which should be co-produced with leaders and activists within the various ethnic minority groups.

A third important area which emerged during the pandemic (once again illustrated in many of our interviews) concerned the *acceleration of online activities,* including everyday social contacts, social events, religious meetings, shopping and medical consultations via telephone or video calls. But questions remain about the possibility of the expansion of digital technology – into areas such as medical care and social support – representing a new form of inequality affecting older people. An ONS (2020) survey conducted around the start of the pandemic found that nearly 40 per cent of those aged 75-plus had never used the internet, and research by Hall et al (2022) suggests that the COVID-19 pandemic did not lead to substantially higher numbers of this group getting online.

Another important finding from work carried out by Age UK (2020) indicates that more than half a million people over 65 are 'lapsed users' of the internet, the reasons including: difficulties in keeping up with changing technology; not having anyone to help when problems arise; health-related issues; and lack of interest and cost. There is some anecdotal evidence that digital exclusion is limiting access to services offered by local authorities (Hall et al, 2022), and that the pandemic may have reinforced this trend. But detailed research is necessary, examining: *the type of groups missing out on digital technology; the support people need to maintain their use of the internet; and the costs as well as the benefits of moving an increasing range of services online rather than face-to-face.*

A fourth area for research concerns the importance of challenging the narrative on ageing and combating ageism. COVID-19 has not only taken a devastating toll on the lives of many older people, it has also exposed a range of discriminatory practices against older adults. The number of deaths (direct and indirect) in care homes from COVID-19, and the delay in recognising the extent of the disaster, illustrate the extent of the crisis in social attitudes towards ageing. Ageism refers to 'the stereotypes (how we think), prejudice (how we feel) and discrimination (how we act) directed towards people on the basis of their age' (World Health Organization, 2021: xv). Such discrimination often intersects with other stereotypes and prejudice, such as those associated with sexism, racism and ableism. As well as discriminatory practices in relation to access to health services, physical isolation measures and strategies for lifting lockdown measures, ageism has also proliferated in news and media coverage of the pandemic, with dominant narratives around ageing centred around stereotypes of vulnerability and passivity. Older people have generally been depicted as a homogeneous, frail group, presenting a burden and risk to other people. Contrary to this discourse, the British Society of Gerontology reminds us of some of the vital, but often ignored, social roles that older adults play in society:

> Older people participate in paid work, run businesses, volunteer, are active in civil society and the cultural life of communities, and take care of family members including parents, spouses/ partners, adult children (especially those living with disabilities), and grandchildren. There are currently more than 360,000 people over 70 in paid work,

including one in seven men between 70 and 75 and one in sixteen women. Almost one million people over the age of 70 provide unpaid care, including one in seven women in their 70s. One in five people aged between 70 and 85, over 1.5 million people, volunteer in their communities. Older adults should not be excluded but should be seen as a vital and necessary part of economic and community life. (British Society of Gerontology, 2020: 2)

The concern, however, is that subsequent waves of COVID-19 infections or future pandemics are likely to further reinforce ageism and intergenerational divisions within communities. The Global Report on Ageism states that 'the ageist narrative around younger and older people runs the risk of pitting generations against each other, as illustrated by the rapid spread of the hashtag "boomer remover" in reference to the virus severely affecting older adults' (World Health Organization, 2021: 25). Research evaluating Twitter communication concerning older adults and COVID-19 found that nearly a quarter of all tweets had ageist or offensive content towards older people (Jimenez-Sotomayor et al, 2020). Given the risk of greater age segregation occurring as a result of COVID-19, it is essential to foster opportunities for greater contact between generations, challenge ageist stereotypes and highlight the diversity of experiences in later life. *Social research has itself an important role to play in highlighting the possibilities of intergenerational exchange, the extent of contacts between generations, and strategies which can promote social cohesion within communities.*

The wider context of precarity

To conclude, we argue that the pandemic must be understood within a wider context of precarity and insecurity. An important argument of this book, developed in Chapter 2, has been that the impact of COVID-19 was increased by pre-existing social inequalities experienced by older people, ethnic minority groups and people living in areas of multiple deprivation. It was further argued that the dominant model of care and support of older people within the health-care system – defined as biomedicalisation – became highly problematic at various points of the pandemic – notably in the treatment of older people in residential and nursing homes, but also in the wider proliferation of ageist attitudes affecting cultural and social institutions.

More generally, we also placed the development and response to COVID-19 within the context of the emergence of a more 'precarious' environment experienced by particular groups of older people, faced with cuts to welfare spending, the upward revision of pension ages and pressures to extend working life. Here, we would support the view put forward by Bonilla that:

Like other forms of crisis and emergency, the pandemic is a socially produced event, driven not by biological forces or natural hazards, but by the deeply-rooted social inequalities that shape our experiences of those hazards to begin with. The pandemic is thus also a disaster in the manner often described by anthropologists and other social scientists: a totalizing and disruptive event that reveals long-standing fragilities and creates new possibilities – both economic and political. (Bonilla, 2022: 420)

The pandemic was especially damaging given its emergence at a time of widening inequalities within societies (Piketty, 2022), and the erosion of collective institutions (such as the welfare state) by market forces. Older people were acutely vulnerable to the effects of COVID-19 – whether from residing in neighbourhoods already damaged by austerity, or living in under-resourced care homes, experiencing under-staffed hospitals, or through the impact of ageist or racist attitudes in access to care and support. But their vulnerability was enhanced precisely because of the weakening of social institutions which can support people during periods of crisis. Streeck refers to the emergence, with neoliberalism, of the '*under-institutionalized*' society, one which fails 'to provide its members with effective protection and proven templates for social action and social existence' (Streeck, 2016: 14, original emphasis). He concludes that: 'Social life consists of individuals building networks of private connections around themselves, as best they can with the means they happen to have at hand' (Streeck, 2016: 42).

But the reality of living in a world with 'more frequent and complex pandemics' (Farrar, 2021: 212), alongside developments such as population ageing, highlight the limitations of an 'under-institutionalised' world and the urgent need to rebuild collective institutions and social structures. Žižek (2020) argues that the response to COVID-19 should be 'new forms of local and global solidarity' and the abandonment of 'market mechanisms to solve social problems' (cited in Horton, 2021: 174). Such comments are especially relevant for challenging the precarious forms of existence experienced by some of the groups interviewed for our research – notably single men living on limited incomes, and ethnic minority groups exposed to racism and inadequate health and social care.

This must involve, as noted in Chapter 9, establishing new or supporting existing forms of collective organisation within local communities through investing in the social as well as physical infrastructure of our communities. In addition, it must also require the rebuilding of the 'welfare' or 'social state' to provide protection for all age groups. As Horton rightly suggests:

Concerns about our health and the risk of further pandemics will trigger debates about the organisation of society. People will no longer see disease as a pathology of the body. We will see disease as a pathology of society. People will demand stronger systems of social protection, especially for the most vulnerable. (Horton, 2021: 184)

But it will be essential that older people themselves play a central role in shaping the debate about the types of infrastructure and resources that will be needed to provide an effective shield against future pandemics. Older people have themselves been victims of COVID-19 (in huge numbers) but they have also demonstrated, as we show in this book, how they found ways to maintain their everyday lives and support others. These are important lessons to build upon and learn from in preparing for future pandemics.

References

Aburto, J.M., Kashyap, R., Schöley, J., Angus, C., Ermisch, J., Mills, M.C. et al (2021) 'Estimating the burden of the COVID-19 pandemic on mortality, life expectancy and lifespan inequality in England and Wales: A population-level analysis', *Journal of Epidemiology and Community Health*, 75(8): 735–740.

Age UK (2020) *Not riding a bike: Why some older people stop using the internet.* London: Age UK.

Alley, D., Liebig, P., Pynoos, J., Banerjee, T. and Choi, I.H. (2007) 'Creating elder-friendly communities: Preparations for an aging society', *Journal of Gerontological Social Work*, 49(1–2): 1–18.

Ayalon, L., Chasteen, A., Diehl, M., Levy, B.R., Neupert, S.D., Rothermund, K. et al (2021) 'Aging in times of the COVID-19 pandemic: Avoiding ageism and fostering intergenerational solidarity', *The Journals of Gerontology: Series B*, 76(2): e49–e52.

Bailey, L., Ward, M., DiCosimo, A., Baunta, S., Cunningham, C., Romero-Ortuno, R., Kenny, R.A., Purcell, R., Lannon, R., McCarroll, K. and Nee, R. (2021) 'Physical and mental health of older people while cocooning during the COVID-19 pandemic', *QJM: An International Journal of Medicine*, 114(9): 648–653.

Bambra, C., Lynch, J. and Smith, K.E. (2021) *The unequal pandemic: COVID-19 and health inequalities.* Bristol: Policy Press.

Barker, D. (2020) Greater Manchester internet exclusion estimate. Greater Manchester Combined Authority, personal correspondence.

Beach, B. and Bamford, S.M. (2014) *Isolation: The emerging crisis for older men: A report exploring experiences of social isolation and loneliness among older men in England.* London: Independent Age.

Beatty, C. and Fothergill, S. (2021) *The impact of the coronavirus crisis on older industrial Britain.* Project Report. Centre for Regional Economic and Social Research, Sheffield Hallam University.

Bengtson, V.L., Elder Jr, G.H. and Putney, N.M. (2012) 'The life course perspective on ageing: Linked lives, timing, and history', in J. Katz, S. Peace and S. Spurr (eds) *Adult lives: A life course perspective.* Bristol: Policy Press, pp 9–18.

Blair, T. and Minkler, M. (2009) 'Participatory action research with older adults: Key principles in practice', *The Gerontologist*, 49(5): 651–662.

Blieszner, R., Ogletree, A.M. and Adams, R.G. (2019) 'Friendship in later life: A research agenda', *Innovation in Aging*, 3(1): 1–18.

Bonilla, Y. (2022) 'Pandemic deja vu', in T. Sugrue and C. Zaloom (eds) *The long year: A 2020 reader.* New York: Columbia University Press.

Booth, R. and McIntyre, N. (2021) 'Covid-related deaths in care homes jump by 46%', *The Guardian* [online], 19 January. Available from: www.theg uardian.com/world/2021/jan/19/covid-related-deaths-in-care-homes-in-england-jump [Accessed 22 January 2021].

Bowlby, S. (2012) 'Recognising the time–space dimensions of care: Caringscapes and carescapes', *Environment and Planning A*, 44(9): 2101–2118.

British Academy (2021) *The COVID decade: Understanding the long-term societal impacts of COVID-19*. London: The British Academy.

British Society of Gerontology (2020) 'Covid-19: Statement from the president and members of the National Executive Committee of the British Society of Gerontology'. Available from: www.ageingissues.wordpress.com/2020/03/21/covid19-statement-from-the-president-and-membersof-the-natio nal-executive-committee-of-the-brit ish-society-of-gerontology/ [Accessed 29 July 2022].

Buffel, T. (2019) 'Older co-researchers exploring age-friendly communities: An "insider" perspective on the benefits and challenges of peer-research', *The Gerontologist*, 59(3): 538–548.

Buffel, T., Handler, S. and Phillipson, C. (2018) *Age-friendly cities and communities*. Bristol: Policy Press.

Buffel, T., Doran, P., Mhorag, G., Lang, L., Phillipson, C., Yarker, S. et al (2021) 'Locked down by inequality: Why place matters for older people during COVID-19', Emerald Publishing Blogs. Available from: www. emeraldgrouppublishing.com/opinion-and-blog/locked-down-inequal ity-why-place-matters-older-people-during-covid-19

Bundy, H., Lee, H.M., Sturkey, K.N. and Caprio, A.J. (2021) 'The lived experience of already-lonely older adults during COVID-19', *The Gerontologist*, 61(6): 870–877.

Butler, J. (2009) *Frames of war: When is life grievable?* London: Verso Books.

Calvert, J. and Arbuthnot, G. (2021) *Failures of state: The inside story of Britain's battle with coronavirus*. London: HarperCollins.

Centre for Ageing Better (2020) 'Homes, health and COVID-19: How poor-quality homes have contributed to the pandemic'. Available from: www.age ing-better.org.uk/sites/ default/files/2020-09/Homes-health-andCOVID-19.pdf [Accessed 28 April 2021].

Christakis, N. (2020) *Apollo's arrow: The profound and enduring influence of coronavirus on the way we live*. New York: Little, Brown Spark

Clough, R., Green, B., Hawkes, B., Raymond, G. and Bright, L. (2006) *Older people as researchers: Evaluating a participative project*. York: Joseph Rowntree Foundation.

Conradson, D. (2003) 'Geographies of care: Spaces, practices, experiences', *Social & Cultural Geography*, 4(4): 451–454.

Corley, J., Okely, J.A., Taylor, A.M., Page, D., Welstead, M., Skarabela, B. et al (2021) 'Home garden use during COVID-19: Associations with physical and mental wellbeing in older adults', *Journal of Environmental Psychology*, 73: 101545.

Cotterell, N., Buffel, T. and Phillipson, C. (2018) 'Preventing social isolation in older people', *Maturitas*, 113: 80–84.

Courtney, K. and Cooper, V. (2021) 'People with learning disabilities are highly vulnerable', *British Medical Journal*, 374: n1701.

Curry, N. (2021) *Beyond Covid-19 wave two: What now for care homes?* London: Nuffield Trust.

Dannefer, D. (2021) *Age and the reach of the sociological imagination: Power, ideology and the life course.* New York: Routledge.

Davis, J. (2022) 'The perfect storm: An NHS in crisis meets the COVID pandemic', in J. Lister and J. Davis (eds) *NHS under siege: The fight to save it in the age of COVID.* London: Merlin Books, pp 44–92.

Di Gessa, G. and Price, D. (2022) 'The impact of shielding during the COVID-19 pandemic on mental health: Evidence from the English Longitudinal Study of Ageing', *The British Journal of Psychiatry*, 221(4): 637–643.

Emmel, N. and Hughes, K. (2010) '"Recession, it's all the same to us son": The longitudinal experience (1999–2010) of deprivation', *Twenty-First Century Society*, 5(2): 171–181.

Estes, C.L. and Binney, E.A. (1989) 'The biomedicalization of aging: Dangers and dilemmas', *The Gerontologist*, 29(5): 587–596.

Fancourt, D., Steptoe, A. and Bradbury, A. (2022) *Tracking the psychological and social consequences of the COVID-19 pandemic across the UK population: Findings, impact and recommendations from the COVID-19 social study (March 2020–April 2022).* London: UCL.

Farrar, J. (2021) *Spike: The virus versus the people: The inside story.* London: Profile Books.

Feagin, J.R., Orum, A.M. and Sjoberg, G. (eds) (1991) *A case for the case study.* Chapel Hill: UNC Press.

Fenge, L.A., Jones, K. and Read, R. (2010) 'Connecting participatory methods in a study of older lesbian and gay citizens in rural areas', *International Journal of Qualitative Methods*, 9(4): 320–333.

Finlay, J., Esposito, M., Kim, M.H., Gomez-Lopez, I. and Clarke, P. (2019) 'Closure of "third places"? Exploring potential consequences for collective health and wellbeing', *Health & Place*, 60: 102225.

Fletcher, J. (2021) 'Chronological quarantine and ageism: COVID-19 and gerontology's relationship with age categorisation', *Ageing and Society*, 41(3): 479–492.

Freedman, V.A., Hu, M. and Kasper, J.D. (2022) 'Changes in older adults' social contact during the COVID-19 pandemic', *Journals of Gerontology: Series B*, 77(7): e160–e166.

Fuller, H.R. and Huseth-Zosel, A. (2022) 'Older adults' loneliness in early COVID-19 social distancing: Implications of rurality', *The Journals of Gerontology: Series B*, 77(7): e100–e105.

Gardner, P. (2011) 'Natural neighbourhood networks-important social networks in the lives of older adults aging in place', *Journal of Aging Studies*, 25(3): 263–271.

Garthwaite, K. and Patrick, R. (eds) (2022) *COVID-19 collaborations: Researching poverty and low-income family life during the pandemic*. Bristol: Policy Press.

Gilbert, S. and Green, C. (2021) *Vaxxers: A pioneering moment in scientific history*. London: Hachette.

GMCA (Greater Manchester Combined Authority) (2017) 'The future of ageing in Greater Manchester'. Available from: www. nws.eurocities.eu/ MediaShell/media/TheFutureofAgeinginGreaterManchester.pdf [Accessed 4 May 2021].

GMCA (Greater Manchester Combined Authority) (2018) 'Greater Manchester age-friendly strategy'. Available from: www.greaterman chester-ca.gov.uk/media/1166/gm_ageing_strategy.pdf [Accessed 12 May 2019].

GMCA (Greater Manchester Combined Authority) (2020) 'Keeping well this winter'. Available from: www.greatermanchester-ca.gov.uk/ media/3842/keeping-well-this-winter-final-19-nov-20.pdf [Accessed 16 May 2021].

gov.uk (2020) 'Scientific evidence supporting the government response to coronavirus (COVID-19)'. Available from: www.gov.uk/government/ publications/sage-advice-on-reducing-the-risk-ofcoronavirus- [Accessed 3 March 2021].

Greater Manchester Independent Inequalities Commission (2021) 'The next level: Good lives for all in Greater Manchester'. Available from: https://www.greatermanchester-ca.gov. uk/what-we-do/equalities/ independentinequalities-commission/ [Accessed 1 March 2022].

Grenier, A. and Phillipson, C. (2023) 'Precarity and dementia', in L. Sandberg and R. Ward (eds) *Critical perspectives on dementia*. London: Taylor & Francis.

Grenier, A., Phillipson, C. and Settersten, R.A. (eds) (2020) *Precarity and ageing*. Bristol: Policy Press, pp 119–135.

Gullette, M. (1997) *Declining to decline: Cultural combat and the politics of mid-life*. Charlottesville: University of Virginia Press.

Gullette, M. (2022) 'American eldercide', in T. Sugrue and C. Zaloom (eds) *The long year: A 2020 reader*. New York: Columbia University Press, pp 237–244.

Hall, A., Money, A., Eost-Telling, C. and McDermott, J. (2022) *Older people's access to digitalised services: A rapid literature review*. Manchester: NIHR: Applied Research Collaboration Greater Manchester.

Hall, S.M. (2019) 'Everyday austerity: Towards relational geographies of family, friendship and intimacy', *Progress in Human Geography*, 43(5): 769–789.

Hammond, M, and Wellington, J. (2021) *Research methods: The key concepts.* Second edition. London: Routledge.

Harrop, E., Farnell, D., Longo, M., Goss, S., Sutton, E., Seddon, K. et al (2020) *Supporting people bereaved during COVID-19.* Cardiff: Cardiff University and the University of Bristol.

Heaphy, B. and Yip, A. (2003) 'Uneven possibilities: Understanding non-heterosexual ageing and the implications of social change', *Sociological Research Online*, 8(4): 1–12.

Heath, S., Chapman, L. and The Morgan Centre Sketchers (2018) 'Observational sketching as method', *International Journal of Social Research Methodology*, 21(6): 713–728.

Hertz, N. (2020) *The lonely century: Coming together in a world that's pulling apart.* London: Hodder & Stoughton.

Hewitt, J. and Kapadia, D. (2021) *Ethnic minority older people, histories of structural racism and the COVID-19 pandemic.* Runnymede Trust. CoDE Covid Briefings.

Highmore, B. (2002) *The everyday life reader.* London: Psychology Press.

Horton, R. (2021) *The COVID-19 catastrophe: What's gone wrong and how to stop it happening again.* Second edition. Cambridge: Polity.

Institute for Fiscal Studies (2019) 'English local government funding: trends and challenges in 2019 and beyond'. Available from: https://ifs.org.uk/publications/14563 [Accessed 15 March 2020].

Irvine, A., Drew, P. and Sainsbury, R. (2013) ' "Am I not answering your questions properly?" Clarification, adequacy and responsiveness in semi-structured telephone and face-to-face interviews', *Qualitative Research*, 13(1): 87–106.

Jimenez-Sotomayor, M.R., Gomez-Moreno, C. and Soto-Perez-de-Celis, E. (2020) 'Coronavirus, ageism, and Twitter: An evaluation of tweets about older adults and COVID-19', *Journal of the American Geriatrics Society*, 68(8): 1661–1665.

Kendall-Taylor, N., Neumann, A. and Schoen, J. (2020) *Advocating for age in an age of uncertainty.* Stanford Social Innovation Review. Available from: www.ssir.org/articles/entry/advocating_for_age_in_an_ age_of_uncertainty [Accessed 12 May 2021].

Kim, H.H.S. and Jung, J.H. (2021) 'Social isolation and psychological distress during the COVID-19 pandemic: A cross-national analysis', *The Gerontologist*, 61(1): 103–113.

Klinenberg, E. (2002) *Heat wave: A social autopsy of disaster in Chicago.* Chicago: University of Chicago Press.

Klinenberg, E. (2018) *Palaces for the people: How to build a more equal and united society.* London: Bodley Head.

Kontopantelis, E., Mamas, M.A., Webb, R.T., Castro, A., Rutter, M.K., Gale, C.P et al (2022) 'Excess years of life lost to COVID-19 and other causes of death by sex, neighbourhood deprivation, and region in England and Wales during 2020: A registry-based study', *PLoS medicine*, 19(2): e1003904.

Lekkas, P., Paquet, C., Howard, N.J. and Daniel, M. (2017) 'Illuminating the lifecourse of place in the longitudinal study of neighbourhoods and health', *Social Science & Medicine*, 177: 239–247.

Lewis, C. (2018) 'Making community through the exchange of material objects', *Journal of Material Culture*, 23(3): 295–311.

Lewis, C. (2020) 'Listening to community: The aural dimensions of neighbouring', *The Sociological Review*, 68(1): 94–109.

Lewis, C. and Buffel, T. (2020) 'Aging in place and the places of aging: A longitudinal study', *Journal of Aging Studies*, 54: 100870.

Lewis, C. and Cotterell, N. (2018) *Social isolation and older black, Asian and minority ethnic people in Greater Manchester*. Manchester: Manchester Institute for Collaborative Research on Ageing.

Lewis, C. and Symons, J. (2017) 'Introduction: Tackling the urban through ethnography', in *Realising the city*. Manchester: Manchester University Press, pp 1–18.

Lindley, S., Ashton, J., Barker, A., Benton, J., Cavan, G., Christian, R. et al (2020) 'Nature and ageing well in towns and cities: Why the natural environment matters for healthy ageing'. Available from: www.ghiadotorgdotuk.files.wordpress.com/2020/01/ghia_report_online_lores.pdf [Accessed 1 February 2021].

Littlechild, R., Tanner, D. and Hall, K. (2015) 'Co-research with older people: Perspectives on impact', *Qualitative Social Work*, 14(1): 18–35.

Lorenz, D. and Dittmer, C. (2022) 'The pandemic's brief disaster utopia', in T. Sugrue and C. Zaloom (eds) *The long year: A 2020 reader*. New York: Columbia University Press, pp 469–480.

Lupton, D. and Willis, K. (2021) *The COVID-19 crisis: Social perspectives*. London: Routledge.

Macdonald, B. and Hülür, G. (2021) 'Well-being and loneliness in Swiss older adults during the COVID-19 pandemic: The role of social relationships', *The Gerontologist*, 61(2): 240–250.

Manchester City Council (2022) *Building back fairer: Tackling health inequalities in Manchester 2022–2027*. Manchester: Manchester City Council.

Marmot, M., Allen, J., Goldblatt, P., Herd, E. and Morrison, J. (2020) *Build back fairer: The COVID-19 Marmot review*. London: Institute of Health Equity.

Marston, C., Renedo, A. and Miles, S. (2020) 'Community participation is crucial in a pandemic', *Lancet*, 395: 1676–1678.

May, V. (2018) 'Belonging across the lifetime: Time and self in Mass Observation accounts', *The British Journal of Sociology*, 69(2): 306–322.

May, V. and Lewis, C. (2020) 'Researching embodied relationships with place: Rehabilitating the sit-down interview', *Qualitative Research*, 20(2): 127–142.

May, V. and Nordqvist, P. (eds) (2019) *Sociology of personal life.* London: Bloomsbury Publishing.

McKenna, K., Williams, J., Humphreys, A., Campbell-Jack, D., Whitely, J. and Cox, K. (2022) *The ageing better programme: Summative report.* London: The Community Fund.

Milligan, C. and Wiles, J. (2010) Landscapes of care. *Progress in Human Geography*, 34(6): 736–754.

Munford, L., Mott, L., Davies, H., McGowan, V. and Bambra, C. (2022) *Overcoming health inequalities in 'left behind' neighbourhoods.* London: All Parliamentary Group for Left Behind Neighbourhoods.

Nafilyn, V., Islam, N., Mathur, R., Ayoubkhani, D., Banerjee, A., Glickman, M. et al (2021) 'Ethnic differences in COVID-19 mortality during the first two waves of the coronavirus pandemic: A nationwide cohort study of 29 million adults in England', *European Journal of Epidemiology*, 36(6): 605–617.

Nazroo, J. and Bécares, L. (2021) *Ethnic inequalities in COVID-19 mortality: A consequence of persistent racism.* London: Runnymede Trust.

Novick, G. (2008) 'Is there a bias against telephone interviews in qualitative research?', *Research in Nursing & Health*, 31(4): 391–398.

Oldenburg, R. (1989) *The great good place: Cafes, coffee shops, community centers, beauty parlors, general stores, bars, hangouts, and how they get you through the day.* New York: Marlow and Company.

ONS (Office for National Statistics) (2019) *The next level: Good lives for all in Greater Manchester – the report of the Greater Manchester Inequalities Commission.* Available from: www.greatermanchester-ca.gov.uk/media/4337/gmca_independent-inequalities-commission_v15.pdf

ONS (Office for National Statistics) (2020) *Internet users UK, 2020.* London: ONS.

ONS (Office for National Statistics) (2021) *Internet users.* London: ONS.

ONS (Office for National Statistics) (2022a) *Coronavirus (COVID-19) latest insights: Deaths.* London: ONS.

ONS (Office for National Statistics) (2022b) *Coronavirus (COVID-19) related deaths by ethnic group, England and Wales.* London: ONS.

ONS (Office for National Statistics) (2022c) *Coronavirus (COVID-19) latest insights: Deaths.* Available from: https://www.ons.gov.uk/peoplepopulationandcommunity/healthandsocialcare/conditionsanddiseases/articles/coronaviruscovid19/latestinsights [Accessed 5 October 2022].

ONS (Office for National Statistics) (2022d) *Manchester population change: Census 2021.* Available from: https://www.ons.gov.uk/visualisations/censuspopulationchange/E08000003/ [Accessed 14 December 2022].

Phillipson, C., Lang, L., Yarker, S., Lewis, C., Doran, P., Goff, M. et al (2021) 'COVID-19 and social exclusion: Experiences of older people living in areas of multiple deprivation', Manchester Institute for Collaborative Research on Ageing.

Piketty, T. (2022) *A brief history of inequality.* Cambridge, MA: Harvard University Press.

Portacolone, E., Chodos, A., Halpern, J., Covinsky, K.E., Keiser, S., Fung, J. et al (2021) 'The effects of the COVID-19 pandemic on the lived experience of diverse older adults living alone with cognitive impairment', *The Gerontologist*, 61(2): 251–261.

Prattley, J., Buffel, T., Marshall, A. and Nazroo, J. (2020) 'Area effects on the level and development of social exclusion in later life', *Social Science & Medicine*, 246: 112722.

Public Health England (2015) *A guide to community-centred approaches for health and well-being.* London: NHS England.

Public Health England (2021) *Wider impacts of COVID-19 on physical activity, deconditioning and falls in older adults.* Available from: www. assets.publishing. service.gov.uk/government/uploads/system/uploads/attachment_data/ file/1010501/HEMT_Wider_Impacts_Falls.pdf [Accessed 13 June 2022].

Raleigh, V. (2022) *Deaths from COVID-19: How are they counted and what do they show.* Available from: https://www.kingsfund.org.uk/publications/ deaths-covid-19 [Accessed 3 October 2022].

Razieh, C., Zaccardi, F., Islam, N., Gillies, C.L., Chudasama, Y.V., Rowlands, A. et al (2021) 'Ethnic minorities and COVID-19: Examining whether excess risk is mediated through deprivation', *European Journal of Public Health*, 31(3): 630–634.

Rosen, M. (2022) 'COVID killed so many of us – now the UK government fears our tears and rage', *The Guardian*, 16 July.

Sachs, J., Karim, S., Aknin, L., Allen, J., Brosbøl, K., Colombo, F. et al (2022) *The Lancet Commission on lessons for the future from the COVID-19 pandemic.* Available from: https://www.thelancet.com/journals/lancet/ article/PIIS0140-6736(22)01585-9/fulltext [Accessed 2 October 2022].

Sassen, S. and Arun, S. (2017) *Manchester: Making sense of the place, its strengths and its future.* Available from: www.theconversation.com/manchester-mak ing-sense-of-the-place-its-strengths-and-its-future-78306 [Accessed 12 July 2022].

Scientific Advisory Group for Emergencies (2020) *Factors influencing COVID-19 vaccine uptake among minority ethnic groups.* Available from: www.gov.uk/gov ernment/publications/factors-influencing-covid- 19-vaccine-uptake-among- minority-ethnic-groups-17-december-2020 [Accessed 12 January 2022].

Seifert, A., Cotton, S. and Xie, B. (2021) 'A double burden of exclusion? Digital and social exclusion of older adults in times of COVID-19', *The Journals of Gerontology: Series B*, 76(3): e99–e103.

Sennett, R. (2020) 'The public realm', in S. Goldhill (ed) *Being urban: Community, conflict and belonging in the Middle East*. Abingdon: Routledge, pp 31–55.

Settersten Jr, R.A. (2015) 'Relationships in time and the life course: The significance of linked lives', *Research in Human Development*, 12(3–4): 217–223.

Settersten Jr, R.A. (2020) 'How life course dynamics matter for precarity in later life', in A. Grenier, C. Phillipson and R.A. Settersten (eds) *Precarity and ageing: New perspectives for social gerontology*. Bristol: Policy Press, pp 19–41.

Settersten Jr, R.A., Bernardi, L., Härkönen, J., Antonucci, T.C., Dykstra, P.A., Heckhausen, J. et al (2020) 'Understanding the effects of Covid-19 through a life course lens', *Advances in Life Course Research*, 45: 100360.

Sherwood, H. (2021) 'Imams across the UK to reassure worshippers', *The Guardian*, 14 January. Available from: https://www.theguardian.com/world/2021/jan/14/imams-mosques-uk-reassure-muslim-worshippers-covid-vaccines [Accessed 20 April 2022].

Simmonds, B. (2021) *Ageing and the crisis in health and social care*. Bristol: Policy Press.

Sridhar, D. (2022) *Preventable: How a pandemic changed the world and how to stop the next one*. London: Penguin Books.

Stafford, P. (ed) (2019) *The global age-friendly community movement: A critical appraisal*. Oxford: Berghahn Books.

Standing, G. (2011) *The precariat: The new dangerous class*. London Bloomsbury.

Statista (2022) 'Number of coronavirus deaths in the US: COVID-19 deaths by age U.S 2022'. Available from: www.statista.com/statistics/1191568/reported-deaths-from-covid-by-age-us/ [Accessed 14 July 2022].

Steptoe, A. and Street, N. (2020) *The experience of older people instructed to shield or self-isolate during the pandemic*. Health ELSA Report. Available from: http://allcatsrgrey.org.uk/wp/download/older_people_2/540eba_55b4e2be5ec341e48c393bdeade6a729.pdf

Streeck, W. (2016) *How will capitalism end*? London: Verso Books.

Sturges, J.E. and Hanrahan, K.J. (2004) 'Comparing telephone and face-to-face qualitative interviewing: A research note', *Qualitative Research*, 4(1): 107–118.

Sugrue, T. (2022) 'Introduction: Preexisting conditions', in T. Sugrue and C. Zaloom (eds) *The long year: A 2020 reader*. New York: Columbia University Press, pp 1–16.

Swift, H.J. and Chasteen, A.L. (2021) 'Ageism in the time of COVID-19', *Group Processes & Intergroup Relations*, 24(2): 246–252.

Sze, S., Pan, D., Nevill, C.R., Gray, L.J., Martin, C.A., Nazareth, J. et al (2020) 'Ethnicity and clinical outcomes in COVID-19: A systematic review and meta-analysis', *EClinicalMedicine*, 29: 100630.

Tarrant, A., Way, L. and Ladlow, L. (2021) ' "Oh sorry, I've muted you!": Issues of connection and connectivity in qualitative (longitudinal) research with young fathers and family support professionals', *International Journal of Social Research Methodology*: 1–14.

Tobitt, C. (2020) 'UK Local Newspaper Closures: At Least 265 Titles Gone since 2005', *Press Gazette.*

UK Commission on Bereavement (2022) 'Bereavement is everyone's business'. Available from: https://bereavementcommission.org.uk/media/jaqex1t5/bereavement-is-everyone-s-business-full-report_1.pdf [Accessed 6 October 2022].

UNECE (United Nations Economic Commission for Europe) (2022) 'Ageing policy in Europe, North America and Central Asia in 2017–2022'. Available from: https://unece.org/sites/default/files/2022-07/Synthe sis%20Report%20including%20Statistical%20Annex_0.pdf [Accessed 15 July 2022].

van Hoof, J., Marston, H.R., Kazak, J.K. and Buffel, T. (2021) 'Ten questions concerning age-friendly cities and communities and the built environment', *Building and Environment*, 199: 107922.

Vindrola-Padros, C., Chisnall, G., Cooper, S., Dowrick, A., Djellouli, N., Symmons, S.M. et al (2020) 'Carrying out rapid qualitative research during a pandemic: Emerging lessons from COVID-19', *Qualitative Health Research*, 30(14): 2192–2204.

Vlachantoni, A., Evandrou, M., Falkingham, J. and Qin, M. (2022) 'The impact of changing social support on older persons' onset of loneliness during the COVID-19 pandemic in the United Kingdom', *The Gerontologist*. https://doi: 10.1093/geront/gnac033

Walsh, K., Scharf, T. Regenmortel, S.V. and Wanka, A. (eds) (2021) *Social exclusion in later life: International perspectives*. New York: Springer Publishing.

Wang, H., Paulson, K.R., Pease, S.A., Watson, S., Comfort, H., Zheng, P. et al (2022) 'Estimating excess mortality due to the COVID-19 pandemic: A systematic analysis of COVID-19-related mortality, 2020–21', *The Lancet*, 399(10334): 1513–1536.

Watkinson, R.E., Sutton, M. and Turner, A.J. (2021) 'Ethnic inequalities in health-related quality of life among older adults in England: Secondary analysis of a national cross-sectional survey', *The Lancet Public Health*, 6(3): e145–e154.

Weeks, J., Heaphy, B. and Donovan, C. (2001) *Same sex intimacies*. London: Routledge.

Whitehead, B.R. and Torossian, E. (2021) 'Older adults' experience of the COVID-19 pandemic: A mixed-methods analysis of stresses and joys', *The Gerontologist*, 61(1): 36–47.

Wiles, J.L., Leibing, A., Guberman, N., Reeve, J. and Allen, R.E. (2012) 'The meaning of "aging in place" to older people', *The Gerontologist*, 52(3): 357–366.

Williams, G., Spencer, A., Tracey, F., Gittins, M. and Arpana, V. (2022) 'Years of life lost to COVID-19 in 20 countries', *Journal of Global Health*, 12. doi: 10.7189/jogh.12.05007

Willis, P., Vickery, A. and Jessiman, T. (2022) 'Loneliness, social dislocation and invisibility experienced by older men who are single or living alone: Accounting for differences across sexual identity and social context', *Ageing & Society*, 42(2): 409–431.

World Health Organization (2018) *The global network for age-friendly cities and communities: Looking back over the last decade, looking forward to the next.* Geneva: World Health Organization. Available from: https://www.who.int/ageing/ publications/gnafcc-report-2018/en/

World Health Organization (2021) *Global report on ageism.* Geneva: World Health Organization.

World Health Organization (2022) '14.9 million excess deaths associated with the COVID-19 pandemic in 2020 and 2021', 5 May. Available from: www.who.int/news/item/05-05-2022-14.9-million-excess-deaths-were-associated-with-the-covid-19-pandemic-in-2020-and-2021

Yarker, S. (2020) *Ageing in place for minority ethnic communities: The importance of social infrastructure.* Manchester: Greater Manchester Centre for Voluntary Organisation.

Yarker, S. (2022a) *Creating space for an ageing society: The role of critical social infrastructure.* Bingley: Emerald Publishing.

Yarker, S (2022b) 'Manchester Urban Ageing Research Group'. Available from: www.micra.manchester.ac.uk/muarg

Yarker, S. and Buffel, T. (2022) 'Involving socially excluded groups in age-friendly programs: The role of a spatial lens and co-production approaches', *Journal of Aging & Social Policy*, 34(2): 254–274.

Yates, L. (2022) 'How everyday life matters: Everyday consumption, everyday politics, and social transformation', *Consumption and Society*, 1(1): 144–169.

Yin, R.K. (1989) 'Research design issues in using the case study method to study management information systems', *The Information Systems Research Challenge: Qualitative Research Methods*, 1: 1–6.

Žižek, S. (2020) *Pandemic! COVID-19 shakes the world.* Chichester: John Wiley & Sons.

Index

www.ingramcontent.com/pod-product-compliance
Lightning Source LLC
Chambersburg PA
CBHW070933030426
42336CB00014BA/2648